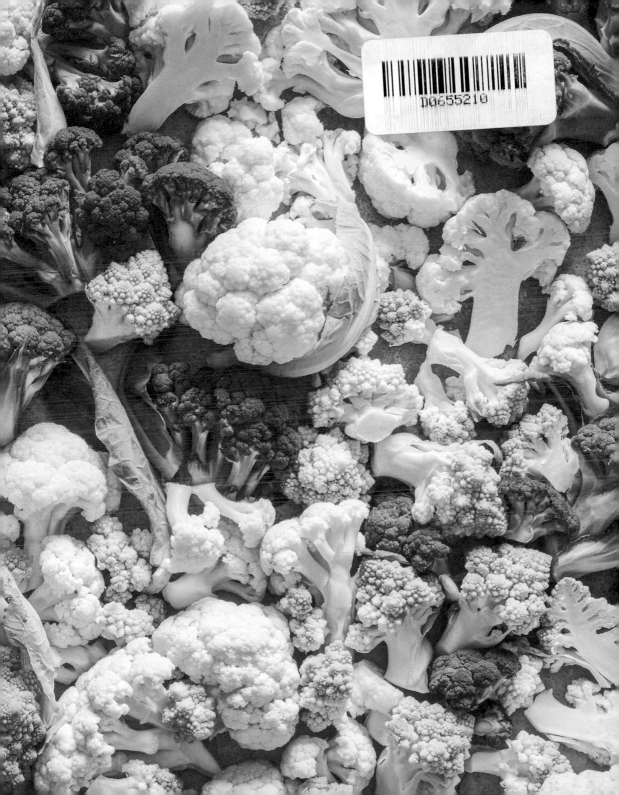

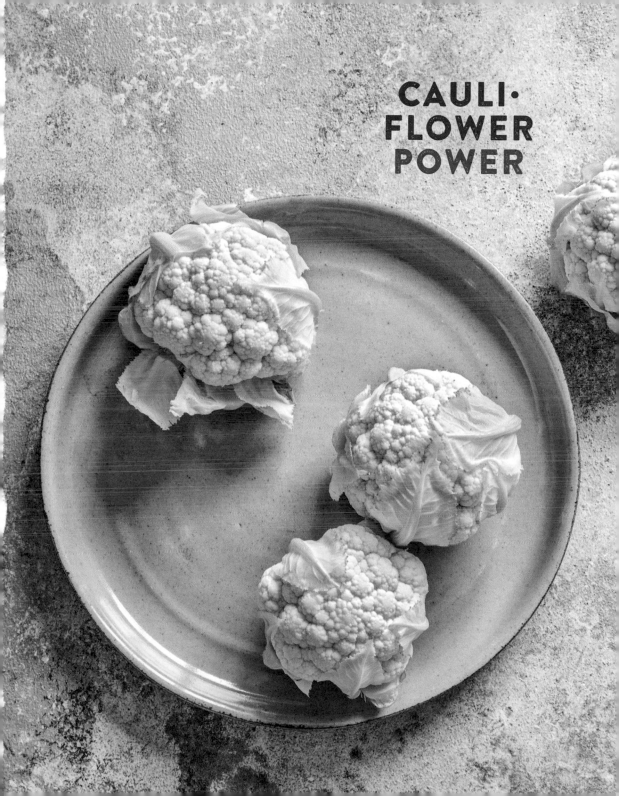

CAULI·
FLOWER
POWER

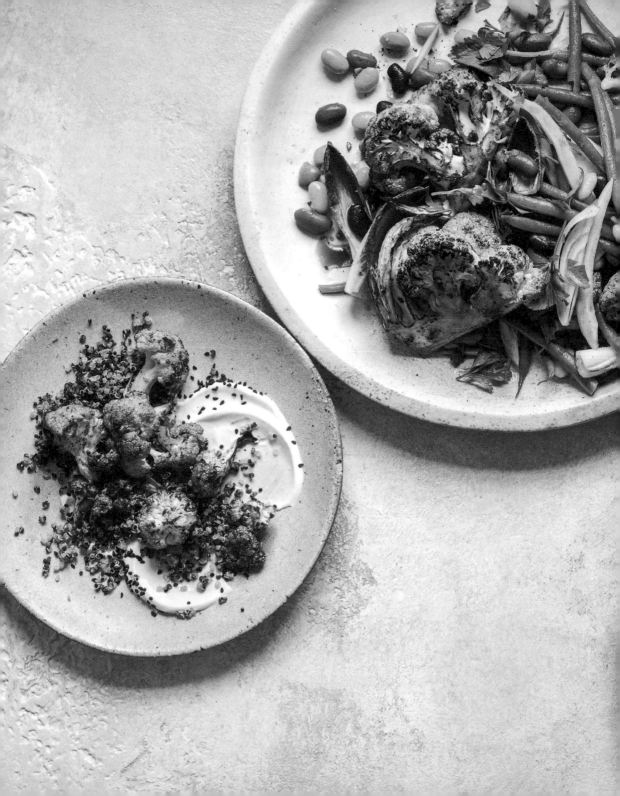

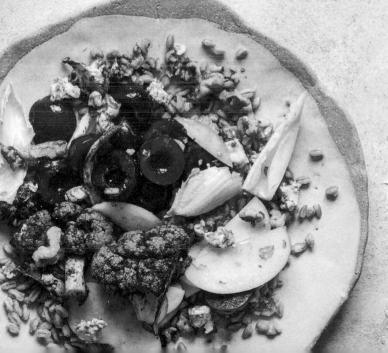
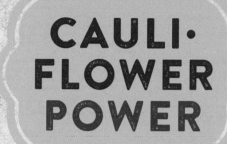

CAULI·FLOWER POWER

VEGETARIAN & VEGAN RECIPES TO NOURISH & SATISFY

KATHY KORDALIS

PHOTOGRAPHY BY MOWIE KAY

RYLAND PETERS & SMALL
LONDON • NEW YORK

Dedication
For Matthew,
my favourite taster!

Senior Designer Sonya Nathoo
Commissioning Editor
Alice Sambrook
Text Editor Kate Reeves-Brown
Production David Hearn
Art Director Leslie Harrington
Editorial Director Julia Charles
Publisher Cindy Richards

Food Stylist Kathy Kordalis
Prop Stylist Olivia Wardle
Indexer Vanessa Bird

First published in 2019
by Ryland Peters & Small
20–21 Jockey's Fields
London WC1R 4BW
and
Ryland Peters & Small Inc.
341 E 116th St
New York NY 10029
www.rylandpeters.com

Text © Kathy Kordalis 2019
Design and photography © Ryland
Peters & Small 2019

ISBN: 978-1-78879-073-4

10 9 8 7 6 5 4 3 2 1

Printed and bound in China.

CIP data from the Library of Congress
has been applied for. A CIP record for this
book is available from the British Library.

Notes for cooks
* Both British (metric) and American
(imperial plus US cups) measurements
are included in these recipes; however,
it is important to work with one set
of measurements and not alternate
between the two.
* Ovens should be preheated to the
specified temperatures. We recommend
using an oven thermometer. If using
a fan-assisted oven, adjust temperatures
according to the manufacturer's
instructions.
* When a recipe calls for the grated zest
of citrus fruit, buy unwaxed fruit and
wash well before using. If you can only
find treated fruit, scrub well in warm
soapy water before using.
* All eggs are UK medium/US large unless
otherwise specified.

CONTENTS

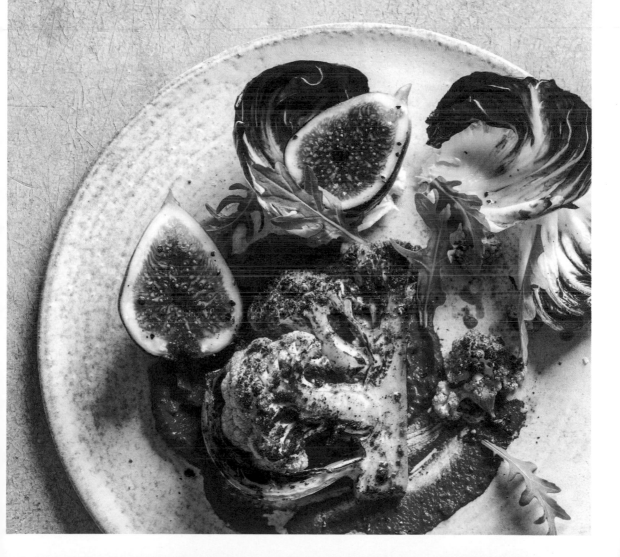

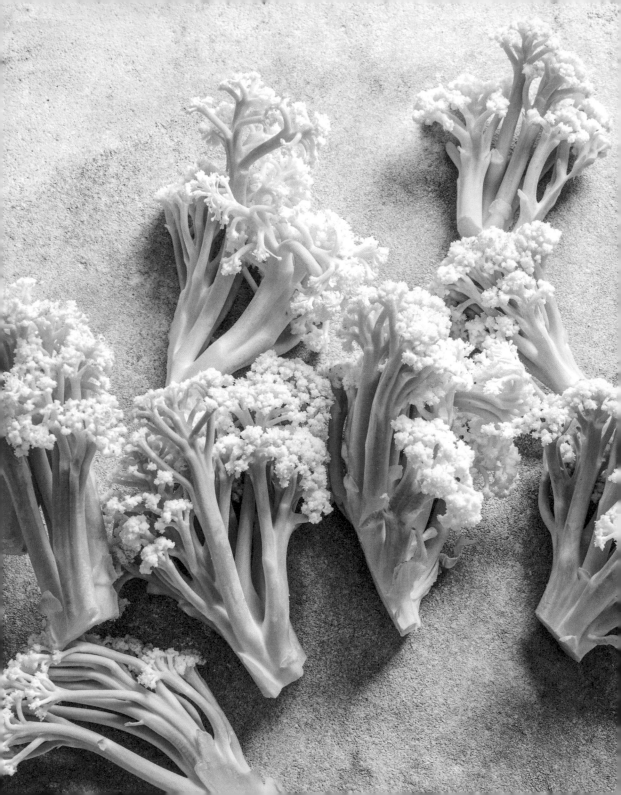

INTRODUCTION

Discover the diverse and delicious super-powers of cauliflower with these stylish and satisfying vegetarian and vegan recipes. Rising from the ashes of its outdated reputation as a forgettable boiled side-dish, cooks everywhere are realizing the potential of cauliflower as a show-stopping centrepiece. When cooked with care, this vegetable is worthy of culinary star status, and this book will teach you how to bring out the best in this charming cruciferous.

The humble cauliflower is available all year around and all over the world. Varieties range from white, to purple, to yellow and now even tenderstem cauliflower, a smaller, sweeter broccoli-cauliflower hybrid (see left).

Cauliflower can be lightly pickled or eaten raw for a super refreshing taste, roasted to bring out a golden, crisp caramelized char, slow-cooked until succulent and tender or blended into something rich and creamy. It is truly one of the most versatile ingredients, able to soak up and seamlessly harmonize with whatever other flavours you throw at it. From Indian to Middle Eastern and Greek to Thai cuisine, cauliflower has a place in kitchens all over the globe.

A master of disguise, cauliflower's substantial texture means that it can be sneakily substituted for less nutritious carbohydrates – it tricks us into thinking we're eating regular rice, pizza dough or mashed potato, and satisfies carb cravings in a much lighter way. A serving of cauliflower also packs a hugely nutritious punch – it's a good source of choline, fibre, protein, omega-3 fatty acids, manganese, phosphorus, biotin, B vitamins and the minerals potassium and magnesium.

In these pages you will find cauli classics with modern twists as well as completely new ideas to try. Sample straightforward recipes in the Simple chapter such as Cauliflower & Butternut Squash Curry or Penne with Olive Oil, Chilli, Cauliflower & Pangrattato. The Fresh chapter features light, zingy dishes such as Cauliflower Carpaccio and Green Goddess Cauliflower Salad, while the Spiced chapter offers fragrant Indian-Spiced Cauli Burgers and Laksa with Cauliflower. In the Rustic section, find soul-pleasing Cauliflower & Potato Hash with Eggs or Freeform Cauliflower Pie with Walnut & Oat Pastry. The Comfort chapter offers Individual Cauli Lasagnes or Cauli Cornbread with Green Chilli & Garlic Butter for those days when you need a little indulgence. Finally, Elegant cauli dishes for entertaining include Double Baked Cauliflower Soufflés and Umami Cauliflower Steaks with Crispy Leeks.

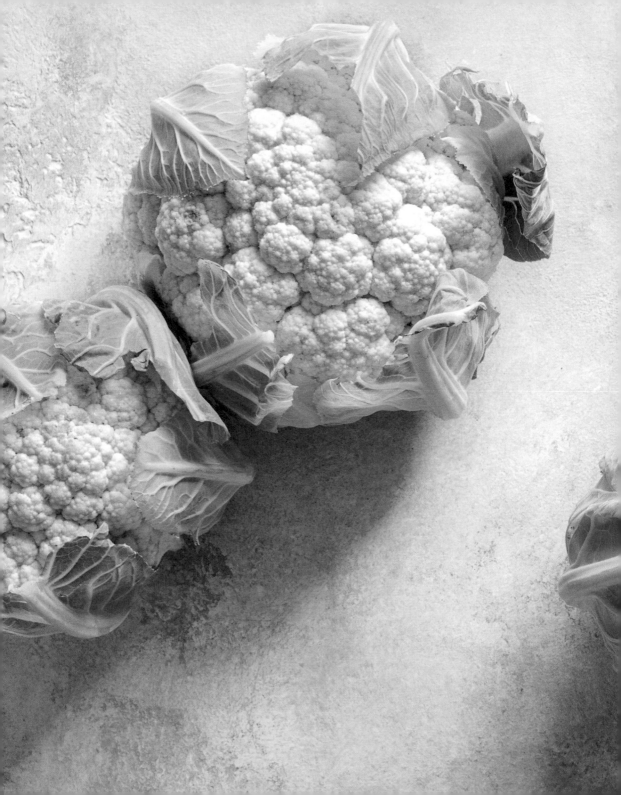

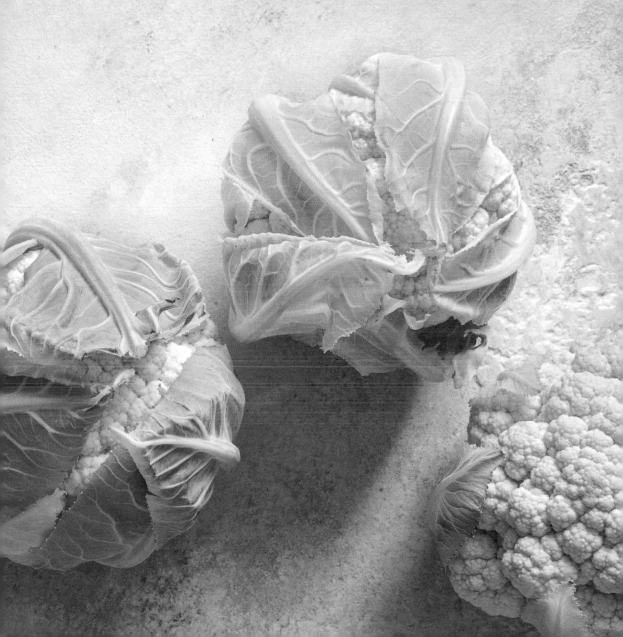

SIMPLE

GREEK ISLAND CAULIFLOWER & TOMATO FRITTERS

Tomato fritters are found all over the Aegean islands, especially in the Cyclades. This version includes the ever-versatile cauliflower, which I find makes them more substantial and satisfying to eat.

SERVES 4 AS AN APPETIZER

5 ripe tomatoes
300 g/10^1/$_2$ oz. cauliflower, grated
4 spring onions/scallions, finely
    chopped
100 g/3^1/$_2$ oz. feta cheese, smashed
50 g/1^3/$_4$ oz. semi-dried tomatoes,
    drained and finely chopped
1 egg, beaten
2 tablespoons freshly chopped
    parsley
2 tablespoons freshly chopped mint
2 sprigs fresh dill
1 teaspoon dried oregano
150 g/generous 1 cup plain/
    all-purpose flour
1 teaspoon baking powder
salt and freshly ground black
    pepper
olive oil, for frying

PARSLEY CAPER SAUCE

2 garlic cloves, crushed
1 large bunch fresh parsley, leaves
    picked
80 g/3 oz. pistachios, finely chopped
100 ml/^{1}/$_3$ cup olive oil
freshly squeezed juice of 1 lemon
2 tablespoons capers, drained
salt and freshly ground black
    pepper

First, prepare the sauce. Add the garlic, parsley and pistachios to a food processor, and process into a chunky mix. Slowly and continuously add the olive oil until you achieve a smooth mixture that holds together. Add lemon juice to taste and the capers. Process again, but keep the sauce chunky. Season to taste and set aside until ready to serve.

For the fritters, cut the tomatoes into four, remove the seeds and discard. Finely chop the tomato flesh and place in a colander with a sprinkling of salt; leave for 30 minutes.

Mix the chopped tomatoes with the cauliflower and spring onions/scallions in a bowl. Add the feta, semi-dried tomatoes, beaten egg and herbs. In a separate bowl, mix the flour with the baking powder and some salt and pepper. Stir the flour mixture into the tomato mixture, until evenly combined and the mixture is firm enough to mould, adding more flour if needed. Refrigerate for 30 minutes.

Place a frying pan/skillet over a medium-high heat and add enough olive oil to cover the bottom of the pan. Dip a tablespoon in some water and spoon out some of the mixture into the hot oil. Repeat this procedure until the surface of the pan is comfortably filled. You should dip the spoon in the water every time, so that the dough doesn't stick on it. Fry in batches for 2–3 minutes on each side, until nicely coloured. Drain on paper towels to absorb the excess oil before serving straight away with the parsley caper sauce.

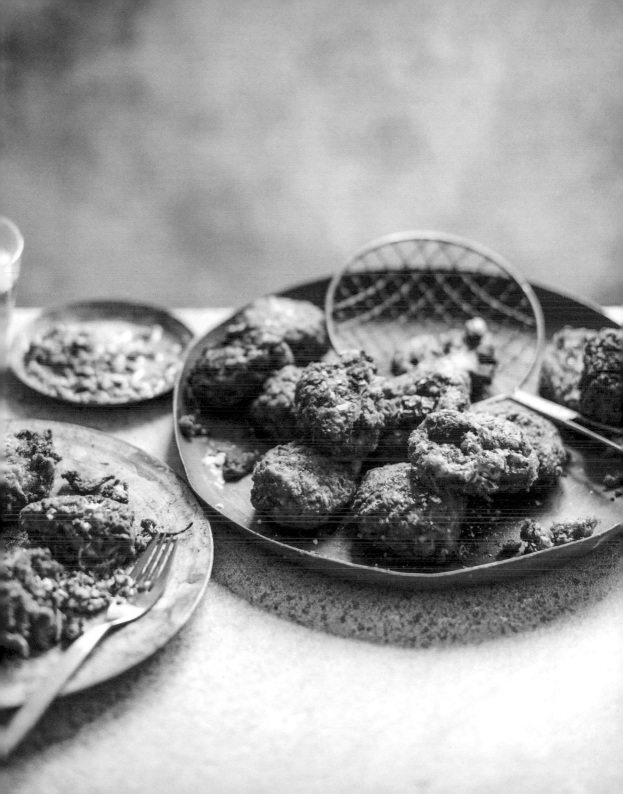

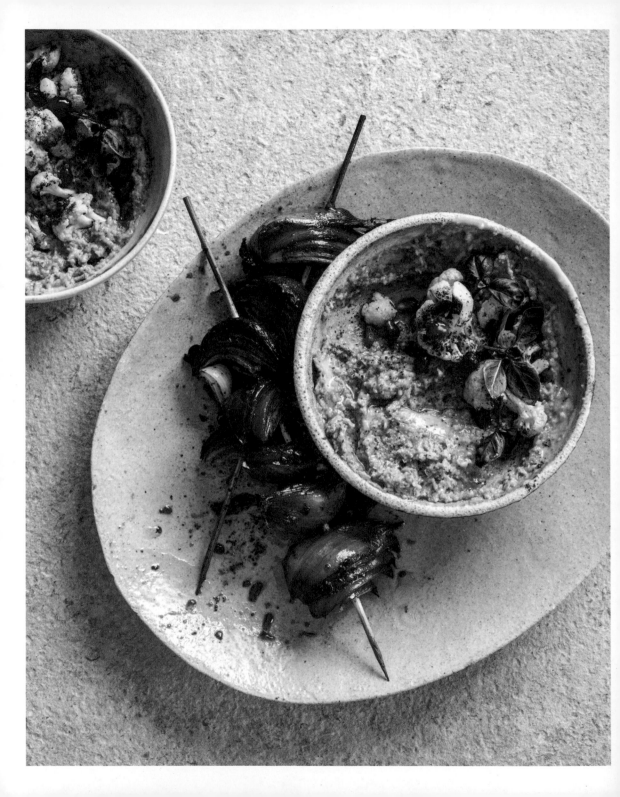

SCORCHED CAULIFLOWER BABA GANOUSH WITH ONION & POMEGRANATE SALAD Ⓥ

This is one of those combinations I could eat all the time. The dip is smoky, creamy and absolutely delicious with the sweet and tart onions.

SERVES 4 AS AN APPETIZER

BABA GANOUSH
2 large aubergines/eggplants (about 650 g/1 lb. 7 oz.)
1/2 cauliflower, cut into florets (about 200 g/7 oz.)
4 garlic cloves, unpeeled
1 teaspoon smoked cumin
4 tablespoons extra-virgin olive oil
freshly squeezed juice of 1 lemon
2 tablespoons tahini
1 tablespoon each freshly chopped mint and flat-leaf parsley
1 tablespoon pomegranate seeds
1/2 teaspoon sumac
purple basil, to garnish (optional)
salt and freshly ground black pepper

SALAD
3 red onions
2 tablespoons vegetable oil
4 tablespoons pomegranate molasses
1 teaspoon maple syrup (optional)
2 teaspoons sumac
1 teaspoon sea salt flakes

baking sheet, lined
2 wooden skewers, soaked for 30 minutes

Preheat the oven to 200°C (400°F) Gas 6.

Blacken the aubergines/eggplants over a gas hob/ring or barbecue/outdoor grill, turning regularly with tongs, until completely charred and collapsed. Allow to cool.

Place the cauliflower and garlic on the lined baking sheet and sprinkle with the cumin. Drizzle with 2 tablespoons of the olive oil and season. Bake in the preheated oven for 10 minutes, then turn and cook for another 10 minutes or until tender and the cauliflower has coloured. Squeeze the garlic out of the skins and set aside with the cauliflower to cool.

Slit the aubergines/eggplants lengthways and scoop out the flesh, discarding the skins. Leave in a sieve/strainer to drain for 30 minutes.

In a serving bowl, stir the lemon juice and 3 tablespoons of water into the tahini until it loosens. Add the mint and flat-leaf parsley and season. Mash the aubergines/eggplants, garlic and cauliflower with a fork (reserving a few cauli florets for garnish), then stir them into the tahini mixture. Top with the reserved florets, pomegranate seeds, sumac and purple basil, if liked. Pour the remaining oil around the edge.

For the salad, peel and quarter the onions, leaving the roots and tips on. Toss the onions in the oil and skewer them. Fry in a very hot griddle/grill pan until charred. Drizzle the hot onions with the molasses and maple syrup, (if using), sprinkle with the sumac and salt flakes. Serve.

CAULIFLOWER OVEN-BAKED TORTILLA

Low-carb and packed with fresh flavours, this tortilla is equally perfect for brunch or dinner. Alternatively, keep it in the fridge for a delicious quick snack. For an extra kick, add a few chillies/chiles to the mix.

SERVES 6

1 medium cauliflower,
    cut into florets
10 UK large eggs/8 US extra-large
    eggs
5 tablespoons olive oil
1/2 bunch dill, leaves picked, plus
    extra to garnish
1/2 bunch coriander/cilantro, leaves
    picked, plus extra to garnish
150 g/generous 1 cup plain/
    all-purpose flour
2 1/2 teaspoons baking powder
1/2 teaspoon ground turmeric
1 1/2 tablespoons black sesame
    seeds, plus extra to garnish
200 g/3 cups finely grated
    Parmesan cheese or vegetarian
    alternative
100 g/3 1/2 oz. roasted red (bell)
    peppers, sliced (jarred work well)
1 large red onion, cut into wedges
50 g/1 3/4 oz. pomegranate seeds
salt and freshly ground black
    pepper

22-cm/9-inch round springform
    pan, base-lined with baking
    parchment and the sides greased
    generously with butter

Preheat the oven to 180°C (350°F) Gas 4.

Place the cauliflower florets in a pan with a teaspoon of salt and cover with water. Bring to the boil and simmer for 15–20 minutes, until quite soft. Drain and leave the florets in the colander for a few minutes to drain further and cool.

Whisk the eggs and olive oil together in a mixing bowl. In a separate bowl, stir together the herbs, flour, baking powder, turmeric, black sesame seeds and Parmesan or vegetarian alternative cheese, then add to the egg mixture, little by little, whisking to remove any lumps. Stir in the cauliflower gently, followed by the red (bell) peppers. Season to taste with black pepper.

Pour the cauliflower batter into the prepared pan and arrange the onion wedges on top. Bake the tortilla in the centre of the preheated oven for 45 minutes, until golden brown and set.

Let cool slightly, then remove from the pan and top with the pomegranate seeds and some extra dill, coriander/cilantro and black sesame seeds. Serve.

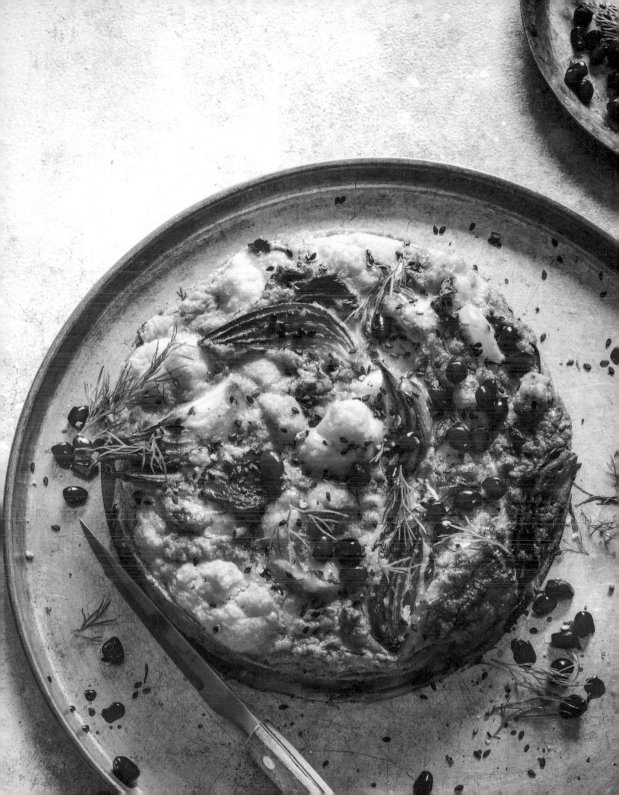

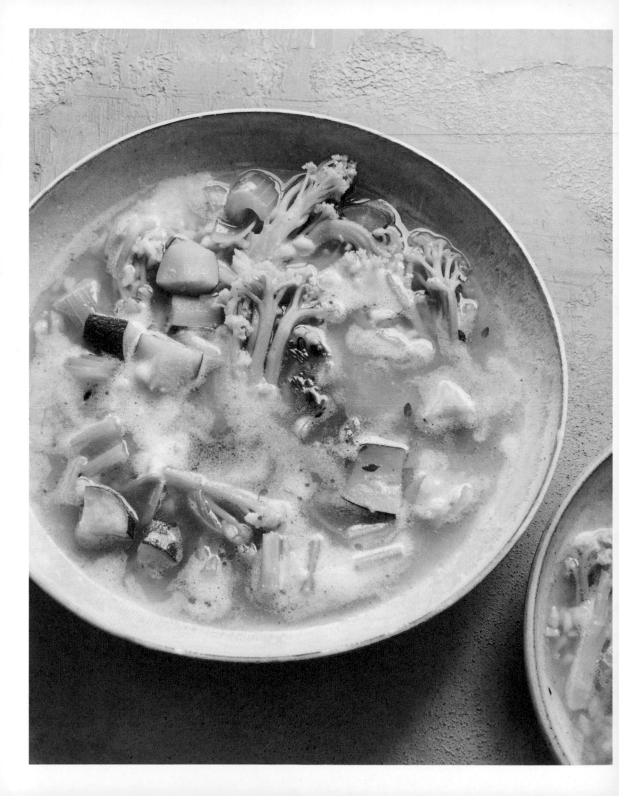

CAULIFLOWER AVGOLEMONO SOUP

The perfect alternative to chicken avgolemono, which is a traditional Greek soup that is thickened with eggs, rice and vegetables. This vegetarian version is soothing, healing and delicious.

SERVES 4

½ onion, cut into large chunks
3 garlic cloves, crushed
2 tablespoons olive oil
2 litres/quarts vegetable stock
1 courgette/zucchini, chopped
½ cauliflower, cut into florets
   or 250 g/9 oz. tenderstem
   cauliflower
100 g/½ cup short-grain rice
1 sprig thyme
2 bay leaves
1 stick celery, chopped
2 eggs
freshly squeezed juice of 2 lemons
salt and freshly ground black
   pepper

Place a deep saucepan over a medium heat, and inside combine the onion, garlic and olive oil. Cook for 5 minutes or until the onion becomes translucent. Add the vegetable stock and bring to the boil. Add the remaining ingredients, except the eggs and lemon juice, to the soup base. Cover and simmer for 25–30 minutes or until the veggies are tender. Season to taste with salt and pepper and then remove from the heat and set aside for a moment.

Add the eggs to a bowl and beat for 4–5 minutes. Mix in the lemon juice. Take two ladlefuls of hot broth from the soup and slowly and very gently pour into the egg froth, mixing to temper the mixture. Don't skip this important step or the eggs will curdle.

Add the mixture back into the soup and stir. Serve with a good amount of freshly ground black pepper.

SIMPLE CAULIFLOWER & BUTTERNUT SQUASH CURRY Ⓥ

This is my favourite mid-week curry! In fact, it's an any-time curry and perfect for when you're in need of rejuvenation. Super-simple, super-tasty and good for both body and soul.

SERVES 4

2 tablespoons flavourless oil
2 red onions, sliced
4 garlic cloves, crushed
4-cm/1½-inch piece each of fresh ginger and turmeric, grated
4 cardamom pods, bruised
1 lemongrass stalk, bruised
2 bird's eye chillies/chiles, halved
2 teaspoons garam masala
1 teaspoon ground cumin
500 g/1 lb. 2 oz. butternut squash, peeled, deseeded and cut into 1-cm/½-inch cubes
4 mini cauliflowers or 500 g/1 lb. 2 oz. cauliflower, cut into florets
2 sprigs curry leaves
400-g/14-oz. can chickpeas, drained and rinsed
400-g/14-oz. can chopped tomatoes
400-ml/14-fl oz. can coconut milk
10 g/½ cup coriander/cilantro, leaves picked
freshly squeezed juice of ½ lime, plus extra wedges to serve
salt and freshly ground black pepper
cooked brown rice and/or vegan naan breads, to serve

Place the oil and sliced onions in a wide, deep saucepan and cook over a gentle heat, with the lid on, for 5 minutes, stirring occasionally.

Add the garlic, ginger, turmeric, cardamom pods, lemongrass, chillies/chiles, garam masala and cumin, plus a splash of water to stop the pan from going dry, and cook the paste for about a minute.

Add the chopped butternut squash and mini cauliflowers or cauliflower florets, plus the curry leaves, chickpeas and canned tomatoes. Add the coconut milk and a little salt and pepper. Stir everything together and bring to the boil, then turn down the heat and cover with a lid.

Cook for 20–25 minutes until the vegetables are cooked through and the sauce has thickened. Add a splash more water if the pan gets too dry.

Add the coriander and lime juice and serve with brown rice and/or vegan naan breads and lime wedges.

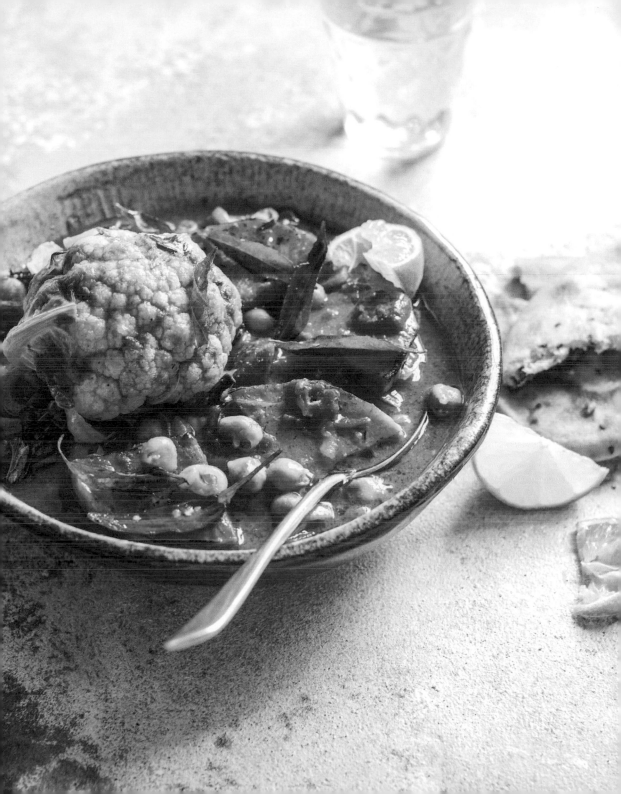

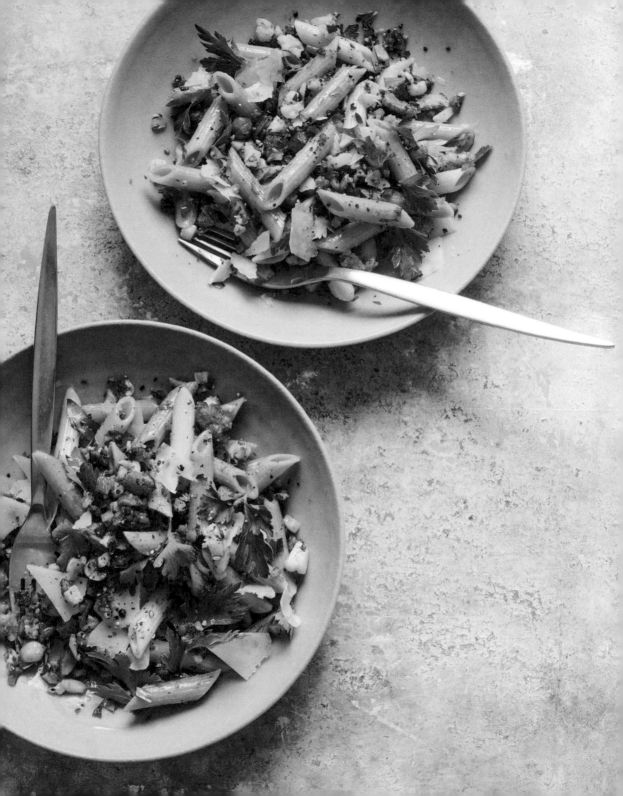

PENNE WITH OLIVE OIL, CHILLI, CAULIFLOWER & PANGRATTATO

Pangrattato in Italian means breadcrumbs. Fried until crisp, it is a perfect topping for pasta. This dish has finely chopped cauli and nuts mixed through, which add even further interesting texture.

SERVES 4–6

2 slices sourdough
knob/pat of butter
½ head of cauliflower, finely diced
2–3 red chillies/chiles, diced
400 g/14 oz. dried penne (or wheat-free alternative)
3 tablespoons good-quality olive oil
100 g/3½ oz. mixed nuts (pine nuts/kernels, almonds and hazelnuts), roasted and roughly chopped
4 garlic cloves, chopped
15 g/¾ cup fresh flat-leaf parsley, leaves picked, plus extra to serve
grated zest and freshly squeezed juice of 1 lemon
salt and freshly ground black pepper
Parmesan shavings or vegetarian alternative, to serve

Toast the sourdough and set aside. Once cool, blitz it in a food processor until you have a rough crumb.

Place the butter, cauliflower and chillies/chiles in a non-stick frying pan/skillet over a medium heat and fry for 8–10 minutes or until golden.

Meanwhile, bring a large saucepan of salted water to the boil, add the pasta and boil until al dente. Drain and set aside.

Add the olive oil, breadcrumbs, chopped nuts and garlic to a separate pan and fry for 3 minutes. Remove the pan from the heat, add the parsley, lemon zest and juice, and some salt and pepper.

Add the penne to the cauliflower and chillies/chiles with half of the pangrattato and toss well.

Place the pasta into serving bowls, sprinkle with the remaining pangrattato, some extra parsley and a generous handful of Parmesan or other vegetarian cheese shavings.

WILD RICE, CAULIFLOWER & GOLDEN RAISIN SALAD

This is my favourite salad ever. Everything comes together in perfect harmony – sweet, tang, nutty, savoury and crunch.

SERVES 4

2 tablespoons olive oil
1 red onion, thinly sliced
1 garlic clove, finely crushed
175 g/6 oz. wild rice
500–750 ml/2–3 cups vegetable
   stock (depending on the rice)
300 g/10$\frac{1}{2}$ oz. tenderstem
   cauliflower
40 g/3 tablespoons butter
30 g/$\frac{1}{4}$ cup hazelnuts, roasted
   and coarsely chopped
30 g/scant $\frac{1}{4}$ cup sultanas/golden
   raisins, coarsely chopped
1 tablespoon sherry vinegar
grated zest and freshly squeezed
   juice of $\frac{1}{2}$ lemon
salt and freshly ground black
   pepper
freshly chopped flat-leaf parsley
   and mint, to serve

baking sheet, lined

Heat 1 tablespoon of the olive oil in a saucepan over a medium-high heat. Add the onion and garlic and fry until tender, about 4–5 minutes.

Add the rice, stir to coat, then add the stock. Season to taste and bring to the boil. Cover with a lid, then reduce the heat to low and cook for 30–40 minutes until the rice is tender and the stock is absorbed. Remove from the heat and leave to stand, covered, to steam for 15 minutes.

Meanwhile, preheat the oven to 200°C (400°F) Gas 6.

Toss the cauliflower with the remaining oil in a bowl and season to taste with salt and pepper. Spread out on the lined baking sheet and roast in the preheated oven, stirring occasionally, until tender and golden, about 15 minutes.

Cook the butter in a saucepan over a high heat, swirling the pan occasionally, until nut brown, about 4–5 minutes. Remove from the heat and stir in the hazelnuts, sultanas/golden raisins, vinegar and lemon zest and juice.

Serve the pilaf warm, topped with the cauliflower, drizzled with the burnt butter and sprinkled with the parsley and mint.

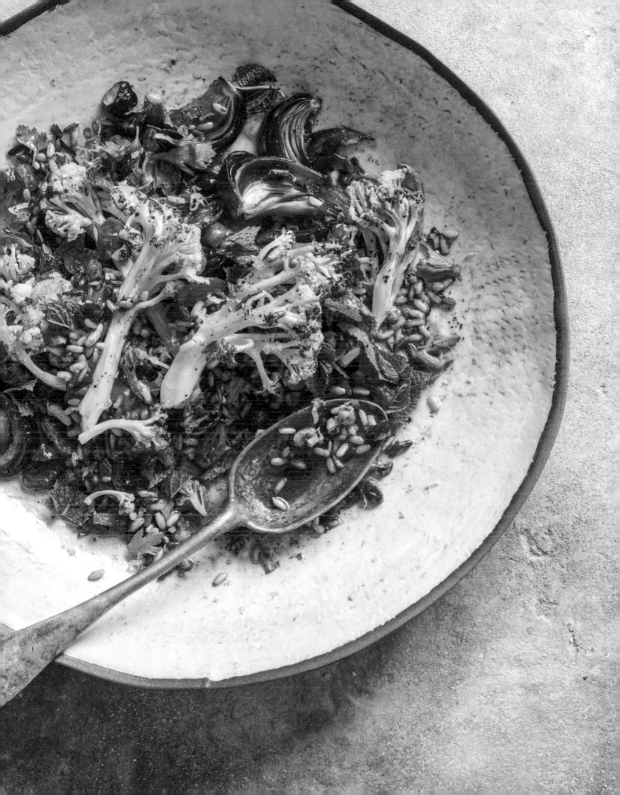

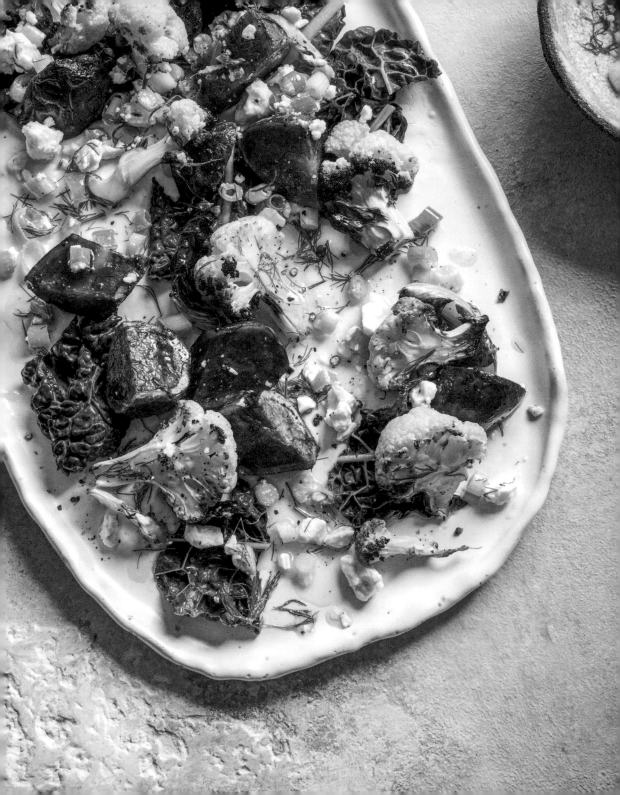

WARM CAULIFLOWER & POTATO SALAD

So many gorgeous flavours together on one platter! This is delicious eaten cold, but is best just warm with the feta, lemon and dill.

SERVES 4

500 g/1 lb. 2 oz. purple potatoes or normal potatoes, scrubbed, skin left on and roughly chopped
60 ml/¼ cup olive oil
350 g/12 oz. cauliflower, cut into small florets
2 garlic cloves, finely chopped
grated zest and freshly squeezed juice of 1 lemon
small bunch dill, finely chopped
100 g/3½ oz. cavolo nero, stems removed and roughly chopped
3 spring onions/scallions, thinly sliced
100 g/3½ oz. feta, crumbled
1 teaspoon dried chilli flakes/hot red pepper flakes (optional)
salt and freshly ground black pepper

Preheat the oven to 200°C (400°F) Gas 6.

In a large, deep baking pan, toss the potatoes with half of the olive oil until well coated. Roast in the preheated oven for 20 minutes, then add the cauliflower and garlic. Season the vegetables well with salt and pepper and stir to make sure they are well coated in oil. Continue roasting for another 20–25 minutes, until the potatoes are cooked through and the cauliflower is starting to colour.

In a bowl, mix the remaining olive oil with the lemon zest and juice, add the dill and set aside.

Put a frying pan/skillet over a medium-high heat, then add the cavolo nero with a few tablespoons of water and cook until just softened. Transfer to a colander to drain any excess water.

Arrange the cavolo nero on a platter and top with the roasted potatoes and cauliflower. Finish with the spring onions/scallions and feta cheese, drizzle with the lemon-dill dressing and sprinkle with dried chilli flakes/hot red pepper flakes, if using. Serve warm.

CAULIFLOWER BRIAM Ⓥ

A Greek-style vegetable bake that is delicious freshly made and warm, but even better the next day served at room temperature. My version includes sweet potatoes, which pair beautifully with the other flavours.

SERVES 6

50 ml/3¹/₂ tablespoons
  extra-virgin olive oil, plus
  extra if needed
200 g/7 oz. sweet potatoes,
  scrubbed and skins left on,
  sliced into rounds
12 cherry tomatoes
3 courgettes/zucchini, sliced into
  rounds
1 large aubergine/eggplant, sliced
  into rounds
1 large onion, sliced into rounds
3 garlic cloves, crushed
250 g/9 oz. sprouting cauliflower
  or normal cauliflower
300 g/10¹/₂ oz. passata/strained
  tomatoes
30 g/1 oz. fresh oregano, leaves
  picked
salt and freshly ground black
  pepper

Preheat the oven to 220°C (425°F) Gas 7.

Add the olive oil, sweet potatoes, cherry tomatoes, courgettes/zucchini, aubergine/eggplant, onion, garlic, cauliflower and passata/strained tomatoes to a large bowl. Sprinkle with the oregano. Season generously with salt and pepper. Combine well with your hands and transfer to a large ovenproof dish. Drizzle with extra oil, if needed.

Bake in the preheated oven for 30 minutes, then turn the oven temperature down to 200°C (400°F) Gas 6. Bake for another 20–30 minutes, or until the top has browned and the vegetables are tender; add a little water if the dish gets too dry. Allow to cool slightly before serving.

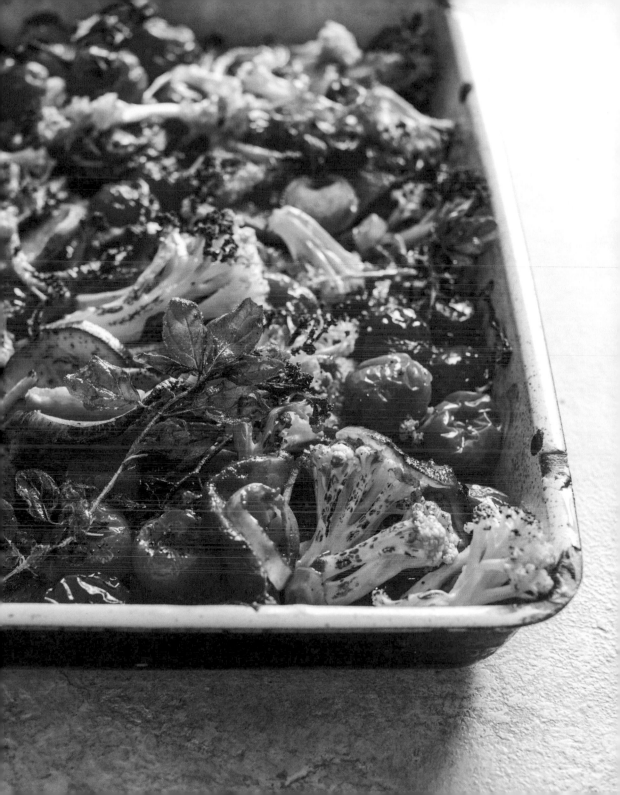

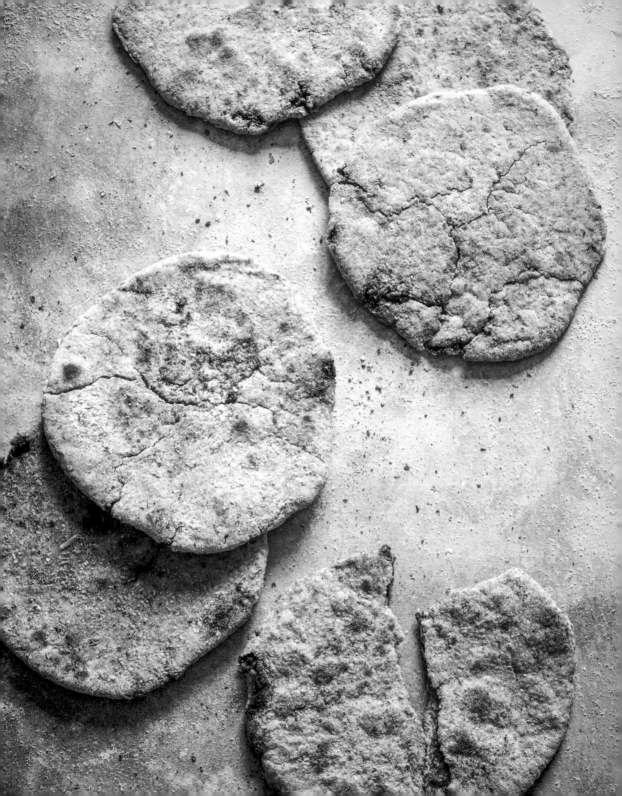

CAULIFLOWER FLATBREADS Ⓥ

These are best eaten on the day you make them... if you can wait until they are all cooked! Have a play with your own flavour combos in the filling – sun-dried tomato paste makes an excellent addition.

MAKES 6

130 g/1 cup wholemeal/
   whole-wheat flour, plus extra
   for dusting
130 g/1 cup spelt flour
1 teaspoon salt, plus extra for
   seasoning
2 tablespoons extra-virgin olive oil
1/2 head cauliflower, cut into florets
freshly squeezed juice of 1 lemon
1 teaspoon coriander seeds, crushed
   in a pestle and mortar
1/2 bunch coriander/cilantro, leaves
   picked and chopped
olive oil, for greasing

Mix together the flours, salt and 1 tablespoon of the extra-virgin oil with 125 ml/1/2 cup water, and knead into a dough. Cover and set aside for 20 minutes to rest.

Blitz the cauliflower to a fine rice-like consistency in a blender or food processor. Dress with the lemon juice and remaining 1 tablespoon of extra-virgin oil, then season with the coriander and some salt, and stir in the chopped coriander/cilantro leaves.

Divide the dough into six balls. Place some wholemeal/whole-wheat flour in a bowl, then dip a ball of dough into the flour and roll it around to coat. Roll out the dough to roughly a 7.5-cm/3-inch disc. Place 1 heaped tablespoon of the cauliflower mixture in the middle and bring the sides of the dough up around the cauliflower. Close and seal by pressing the dough together once again, creating a dough ball. Dip again in the flour, covering the ball, then roll it out to about 13 cm/5 inches thick, without too much mixture spilling out.

Place a frying pan/skillet over a medium-high heat, wipe the base with olive oil – just enough to grease the pan – and cook the flatbreads in batches for 5 minutes on each side until cooked through. Serve warm.

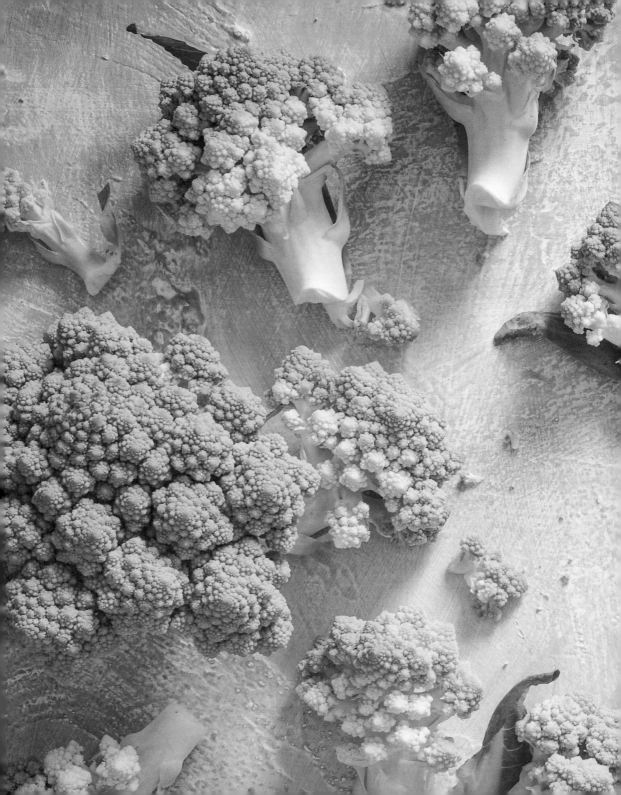

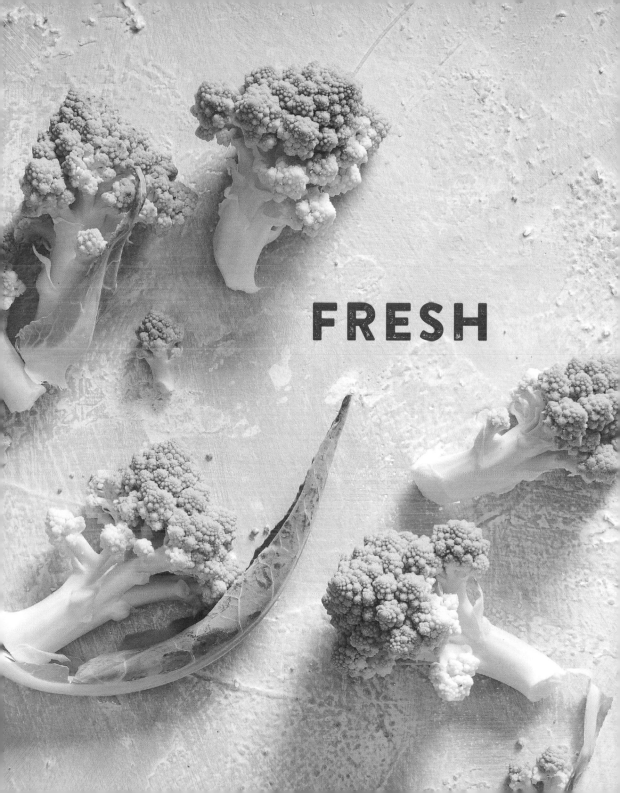

FRESH

CAULIFLOWER HUMMUS WITH QUICK MUSTARD PICKLE ⓥ

The earthiness of the cauliflower hummus here goes perfectly with the tangy, crisp mustard-spiked pickles. Served together with fresh vegetables and/or flatbreads, it makes a great, light mezze spread.

SERVES 4 AS AN APPETIZER

QUICK MUSTARD PICKLE
3 tablespoons apple cider vinegar
3 tablespoons English mustard
1/4 teaspoon ground turmeric
2 garlic cloves, crushed
1 tablespoon mustard seeds
1 tablespoon white sugar
1 teaspoon salt
1–2 mini cucumber(s), thinly
   sliced into rounds
1 red (bell) pepper, diced
1 small cauliflower, cut into
   very small florets
1 large red onion, thinly sliced

CAULIFLOWER HUMMUS
600 g/1 lb. 5 oz. cauliflower
1 teaspoon ground cumin
400-g/14-oz. can chickpeas,
   drained and rinsed
2 garlic cloves, peeled
80 ml/1/3 cup tahini
60 ml/1/4 cup lemon juice
60 ml/1/4 cup olive oil, plus extra
   for drizzling
60 ml/1/4 cup warm water
salt and ground black pepper
1 teaspoon each cumin and
   coriander seeds, toasted, to serve

For the pickle, put the vinegar, English mustard, turmeric, garlic, mustard seeds, sugar, salt and 1 tablespoon of water in a large, non-reactive saucepan. Gently bring to the boil until little bubbles form around the edge of the pan.

Add the vegetables and stir well to coat them in the liquid, then remove from the heat. Press the vegetables into the liquid, then leave to pickle for 1 hour, stirring occasionally. When cool, drain and discard half the liquid and serve immediately with the remaining pickling liquid, or store in a sterilized jar and chill until needed.

Preheat the oven to 200°C (400°F) Gas 6.

For the hummus, place the cauliflower florets on a baking sheet and drizzle with oil. Sprinkle with the cumin and roast in the preheated oven for 25 minutes or until tender. Set aside to cool slightly.

Transfer the cauliflower mixture to a food processor. Add most of the chickpeas (reserving about 50 g/1/3 cup to garnish), the garlic, tahini, lemon juice, olive oil and water. Season and process until smooth.

Serve topped with the reserved chickpeas, drizzled with a little extra olive oil and sprinkled with the toasted cumin and coriander seeds. Perfect with the mustard pickle and some vegetable crudités and/or flatbreads.

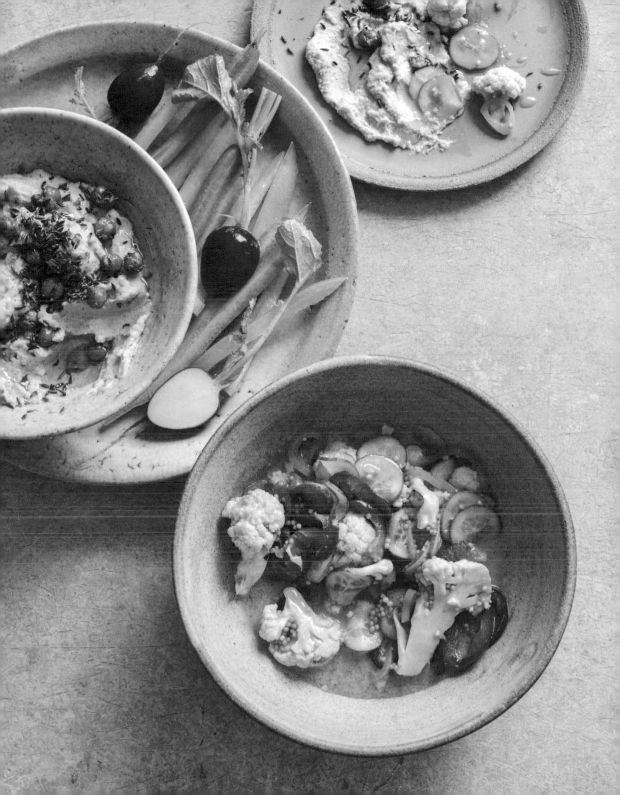

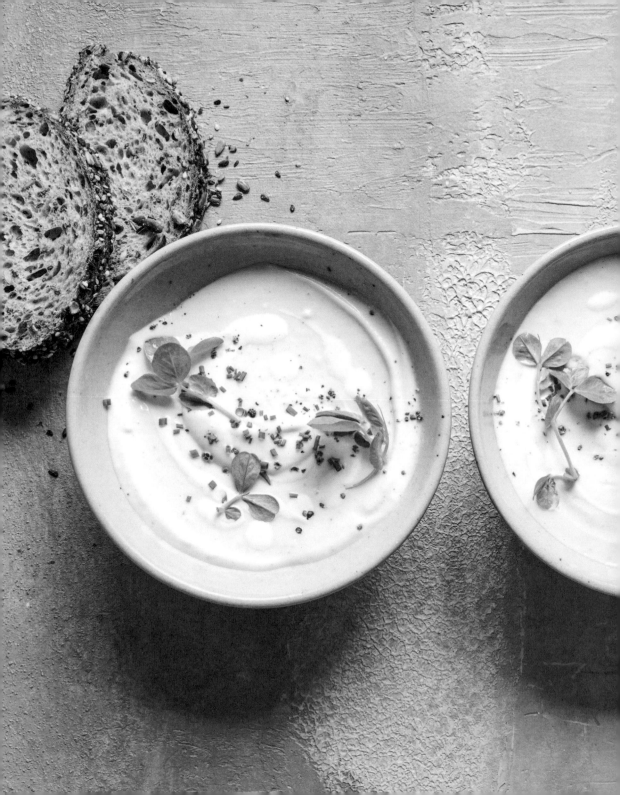

CREAM OF CAULIFLOWER SOUP ⓥ

Vegan heaven in a bowl! This dreamy plant-based soup contains nutritional yeast which gives a deliciously savoury, cheesy flavour without the use of dairy.

SERVES 4

2 tablespoons extra-virgin
  olive oil
4 garlic cloves, crushed
1 onion, chopped
1 cauliflower, cut into florets
1 potato, peeled and chopped
500 ml/2 cups vegetable stock
250 ml/1 cup plant-based milk,
  unsweetened
4 tablespoons nutritional yeast
  (or to taste)
salt and freshly ground black
  pepper

TO FINISH
1 tablespoon oat cream
  or dairy-free cream
handful of chives, finely snipped
handful of pea shoots
crushed green peppercorns

Heat the oil in a large pan and add the garlic and onion. Cook over a medium-high heat until golden brown. Add the cauliflower, potato, stock and milk and bring to the boil. Cook over a medium-high heat for about 15–20 minutes or until the cauliflower is soft.

Add the nutritional yeast and some salt and pepper, and blend until smooth using a hand-held blender.

Serve with a swirl of oat cream and a sprinkling of snipped chives, fresh pea shoots and crushed green peppercorns.

TURMERIC TAHINI CAULI FRITTERS WITH GINGER SALAD

For me, the perfect way to eat these fritters is with this gingery fresh salad. The dressing cuts through the oil of the fritters.

SERVES 4 TO SHARE

½ large cauliflower, cut into florets
60 g/scant ½ cup plain/
    all-purpose flour
1 teaspoon baking powder
2 tablespoons tahini
½ teaspoon ground turmeric
½ teaspoon dried chilli flakes/hot
    red pepper flakes
2 eggs
salt and freshly ground black
    pepper
about 600 ml/2½ cups vegetable
    oil, for deep-frying

GINGER SALAD
15 g/½ oz. piece fresh ginger, peeled
    and cut into julienne
1 tablespoon red wine vinegar
½ teaspoon soft brown sugar
60 ml/¼ cup olive oil
100 g/3½ oz. frisée, preferably pale
    inner leaves (from 1 large head)
salt and freshly ground black
    pepper

Place the cauliflower into a pan of boiling water and cook for 5–7 minutes or until just tender. Don't let it go soggy, slightly undercooked is great, because you want the fritters to have a bit of texture.

Drain and rinse the florets under cold water to stop the cooking process, and pat dry with a paper towel. Chop them into smallish chunks and place in a bowl.

Sift the flour and baking powder into a mixing bowl and add the tahini, turmeric and chilli flakes/hot red pepper flakes. Season. Make a well in the centre and drop in the eggs. Slowly mix with a wooden spoon until incorporated and most of the lumps have gone. Fold in the cauliflower florets and coat them thoroughly in the batter.

Heat the oil for deep-frying in a deep-sided pan until hot. It is at the correct temperature when you drop in a piece of bread and it bubbles instantly.

Take a tablespoonful of the cauliflower mix and slide it into the hot oil, using another spoon to push the mix off if it helps. Always work away from you when deep-frying. Fry the fritters in batches until golden brown, then remove from the oil. Place on paper towels to drain and sprinkle with salt.

For the salad, whisk together the ginger, red wine vinegar, brown sugar and olive oil in a small bowl, season to taste and set aside. Put the salad leaves in a bowl, drizzle with the dressing and toss to combine. Serve with the warm fritters.

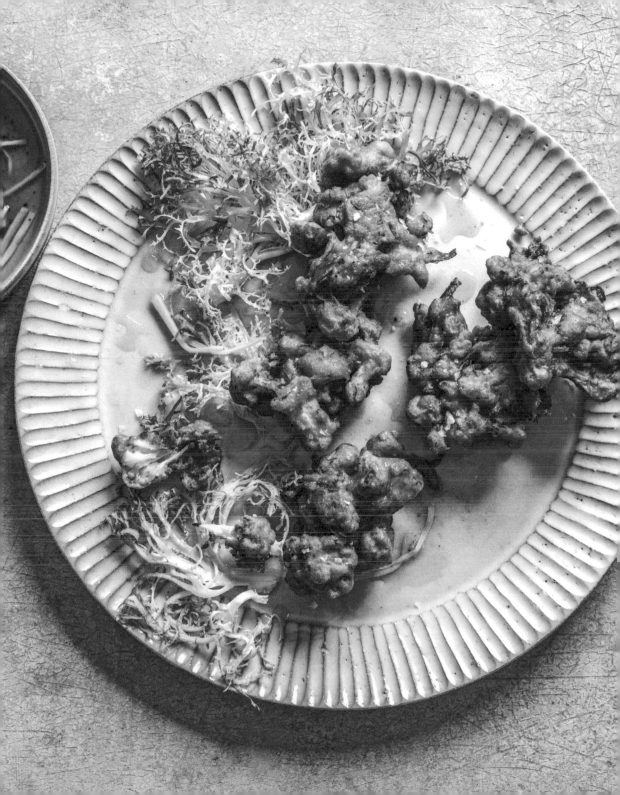

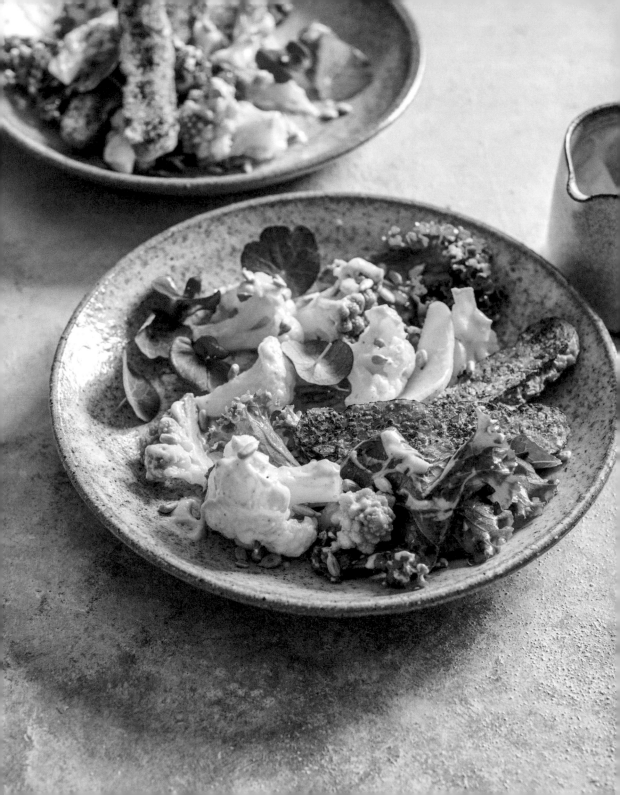

GREEN GODDESS CAULIFLOWER SALAD WITH TEMPEH ⓥ

This is one of those good-for-your-body-and-soul salads. Personally, I prefer to quickly blanch the veg, still leaving a lot of bite, but you can also combine the ingredients raw if you prefer.

SERVES 2 GENEROUSLY

200 g/7 oz. kale, destemmed, chopped, blanched and refreshed
200 g/7 oz. cauliflower, cut into florets, blanched and refreshed
150 g/5½ oz. Romanesco broccoli, cut into florets, blanched and refreshed
60 g/scant ½ cup sunflower seeds, roasted
1 pear, cored and sliced
1 tablespoon olive oil
200 g/7 oz. tempeh, sliced into 8 thin strips
edible flowers, to garnish (optional)

CREAMY AVOCADO MINT DRESSING

150 g/5½ oz. silken tofu
1 ripe avocado, peeled and pitted
large handful of mint, leaves picked
freshly squeezed juice of ½ lemon
½ tablespoon maple syrup
1 teaspoon apple cider vinegar
1 garlic clove, crushed
¼ teaspoon ground ginger
salt and freshly ground black pepper

In a blender or high-speed food processor, blend all of the avocado mint dressing ingredients until smooth and creamy. Season to taste.

In a large bowl, take 60 ml/¼ cup of your dressing and massage it into the kale.

Divide the kale between two bowls and top with the cauliflower florets, Romanesco broccoli florets, sunflower seeds and pear slices – dividing each ingredient evenly between the bowls.

Heat the olive oil in a large frying pan/skillet over a medium-high heat and add the tempeh slices. Cook the tempeh on each side for a few minutes until golden brown and slightly caramelized.

Add the tempeh to each salad and top with more avocado mint dressing.

LEMON & OREGANO ROASTED CAULIFLOWER WITH ALMOND YOGURT DRESSING

This would be a perfect veggie replacement for a Sunday roast chicken. Serve the charred, tender cauli straight from the pan, drizzled with the almond sauce. The juices can be mopped up with flatbreads.

SERVES 2

1 head of cauliflower, leaves left on
4 tablespoons olive oil
3 garlic cloves, crushed and then mashed into a paste
1 teaspoon dried oregano
3 sprigs fresh oregano, leaves picked
1 lemon
salt and freshly ground black pepper

ALMOND SAUCE
100 g/1 cup ground almonds
100 g/$\frac{1}{2}$ cup minus $\frac{1}{2}$ tablespoon Greek yogurt
pinch of ground sumac
pinch of ground nutmeg
grated zest and freshly squeezed juice of $\frac{1}{2}$ lemon

TO SERVE
50 g/1$\frac{3}{4}$ oz. roasted almonds, coarsely chopped
fresh mint and oregano leaves
pinch of dried rose petals
pinch of ground sumac

Preheat the oven to 180°C (350°F) Gas 4.

Place the cauliflower in a roasting tray or a cast-iron pan and rub all over with 1 tablespoon of the olive oil and the crushed garlic paste. Season with the dried and fresh oregano and some salt and pepper. Halve the lemon and add this to the pan. Cover with foil and roast in the preheated oven for 1 hour 20 minutes, removing the foil for the last 20 minutes until the cauliflower is tender and dark golden brown; any charred parts will add to the flavour.

Meanwhile, make the almond sauce. Place the ground almonds in a saucepan with 150 ml/$\frac{2}{3}$ cup water and a tablespoon of the remaining olive oil. Warm through over a low heat for about 5 minutes or until the almonds just start to swell (this makes them easier to blend). Pour the almond mixture into a blender and process to a smooth sauce, then season to taste and mix in the yogurt, sumac, nutmeg and lemon zest and juice.

Remove the cauliflower from the oven and dress simply with the remaining 2 tablespoons of olive oil and juice from the roasted lemon. Scatter over the roasted almonds, fresh herbs, rose petals and sumac and serve with the almond sauce on the side.

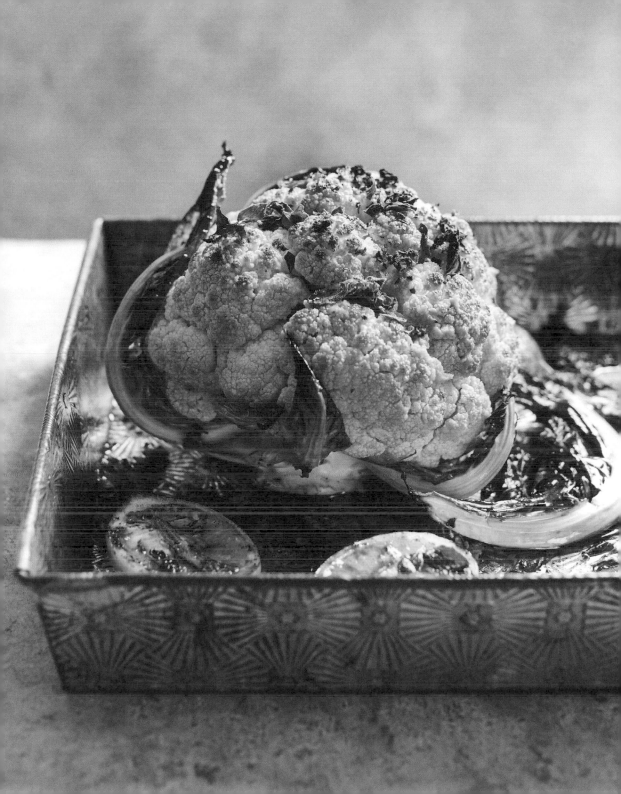

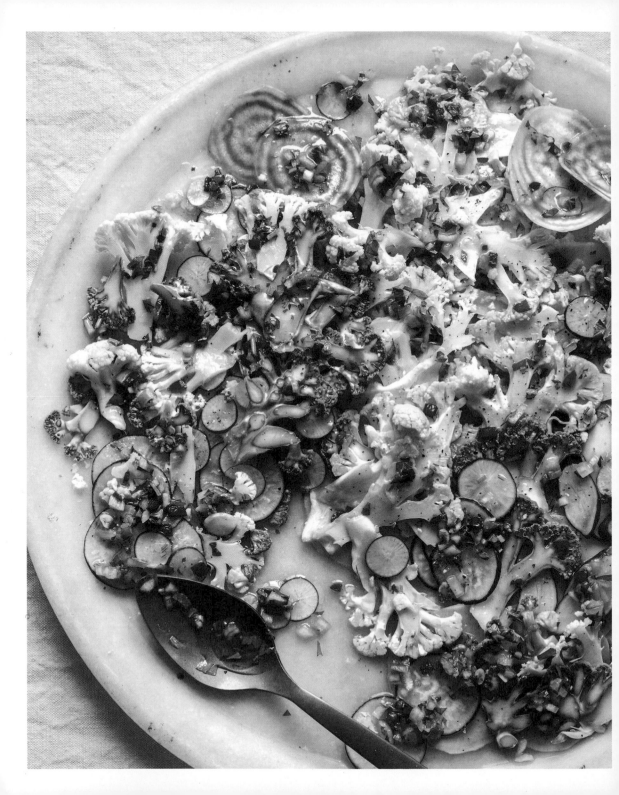

CAULIFLOWER CARPACCIO ⓥ

This is a wonderfully light and refreshing dish. Be sure to generously dress the thinly sliced cauliflower and other vegetables at least 20 minutes before serving, which will give the flavours a chance to meld and let the vegetables soften slightly, leaving some bite.

SERVES 4–6 AS A SHARING PLATTER

200 g/7 oz. cauliflower florets in mixed colours
1 orange or candy striped beetroot/beet, washed and peeled
6 radishes, washed
1 small kohlrabi, peeled
1 small pear, peeled and cored

DRESSING

1 shallot, peeled
50 ml/3$^{1}/_{2}$ tablespoons extra-virgin olive oil
1 red chilli/chile, deseeded and finely chopped
1 garlic clove, finely chopped
1 tablespoon freshly chopped parsley
freshly squeezed juice of 1$^{1}/_{2}$ lemons
freshly squeezed juice of 1$^{1}/_{2}$ limes
1 tablespoon soy sauce
1 tablespoon maple syrup
salt and freshly ground black pepper

For the dressing, thinly slice the shallot on a mandoline into thin rounds and place into a bowl.

Mix in the olive oil, red chilli/chile, garlic, parsley, lemon and lime juices, soy sauce and maple syrup and season well. Whisk again and set to one side.

Using a very sharp knife and a very steady hand or, preferably, a mandoline, slice each of the vegetables and the pear thinly. Try to vary the shapes, for example, slicing some vegetables lengthways. Arrange the vegetables and pear across a serving plate, then drizzle with 3 tablespoons of the dressing.

Allow to sit for at least 20 minutes before serving to allow the flavours to infuse. Serve with the remaining dressing.

MIXED BRASSICA SALAD WITH HORSERADISH & LEMON DRESSING

Pure freshness on a plate with a fiery kick from the horseradish. The most important thing to remember here is to dress this simple salad well in advance of serving to give the vegetables time to soften slightly.

SERVES 4–6

100 g/²⁄₃ cup fresh peas
1 cauliflower, thinly sliced
200 g/7 oz. cabbage, shredded
200 g/7 oz. Brussels sprouts, shredded
150 g/5¹⁄₂ oz. small radishes, thinly sliced lengthways
20 g/1 cup each (loosely packed) mint and flat-leaf parsley, torn, plus extra to garnish
1 long green chilli/chile, deseeded and finely chopped
80 g/1¹⁄₂ cups finely grated Parmesan cheese (optional) or vegetarian alternative
salt and freshly ground black pepper

HORSERADISH LEMON DRESSING

fresh horseradish, grated, to taste
100 ml/¹⁄₃ cup extra-virgin olive oil
50 ml/3¹⁄₂ tablespoons freshly squeezed lemon juice
salt and freshly ground black pepper

Blanch the peas in boiling water for 1–2 minutes or until bright green, then drain, refresh, drain again and set aside until needed.

For the horseradish lemon dressing, whisk all the ingredients together in a bowl, season to taste and set aside.

Combine the cauliflower, cabbage, Brussels sprouts, radishes, herbs, chilli/chile and half the Parmesan or vegetarian alternative (if using) in a large bowl and toss to combine. Add the lemon dressing, season to taste and mix until the cabbage begins to wilt.

Serve the salad scattered with the peas, the remaining cheese (if using) and extra herbs.

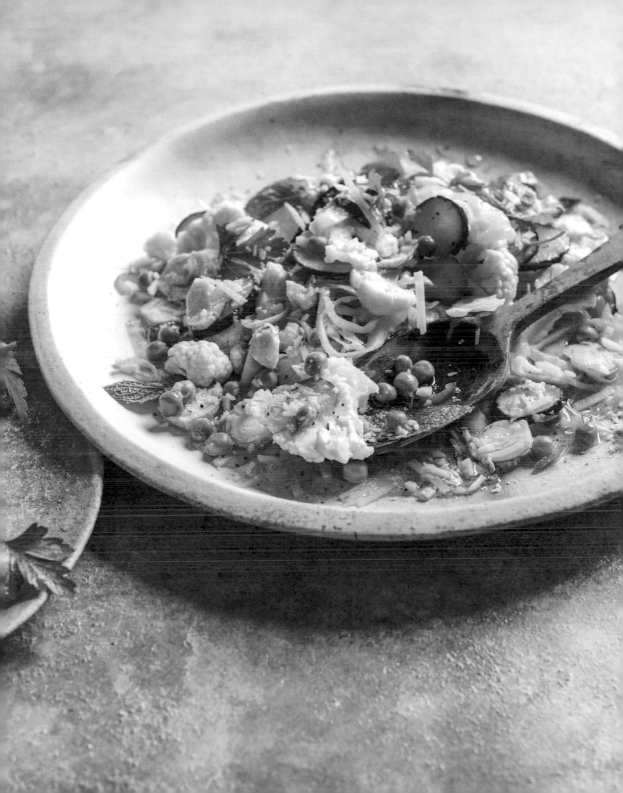

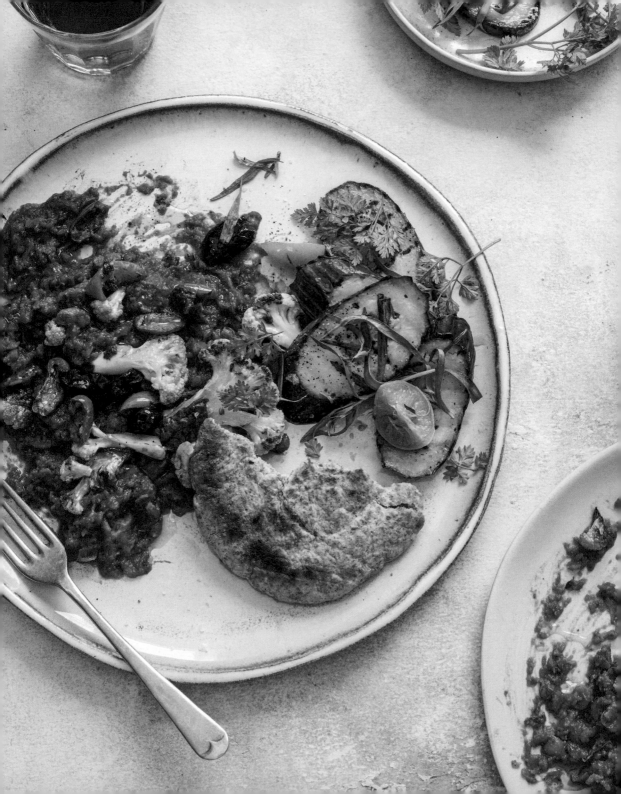

CAULIFLOWER FAVA WITH CRISPY OLIVES & GRIDDLED CUCUMBER Ⓥ

Another twist on a Greek island recipe, and so absolutely versatile. You can serve it as a dip, a side dish, or snack on it to your heart's content.

SERVES 4

300 g/10½ oz. cauliflower florets
200 g/1 cup plus 2 tablespoons
   yellow split peas, well-rinsed
4 tablespoons olive oil
1 bay leaf
1 onion, finely chopped
2 cloves garlic, crushed
1 tablespoon dried oregano
1 tablespoon tomato purée/paste
1 tablespoon sun-dried tomato
   paste
1 litre/quart vegetable stock
1 tablespoon sherry vinegar
1 teaspoon salt (more as needed)
   and freshly ground black pepper

GRIDDLED CUCUMBER

1 cucumber
2 tablespoons olive oil
2 sprigs fresh tarragon, leaves
   picked and chopped
3 sprigs fresh chervil, leaves picked
½ bunch fresh chives, finely
   chopped
½ preserved lemon, thinly sliced

TO SERVE

reserved cauliflower (thinly sliced)
1 tablespoon pitted green or black
   olives, rinsed and sliced
pitta breads

Reserve 100 g/3½ oz. of the cauliflower, but place the rest in a heavy-based saucepan with the yellow split peas and 1 tablespoon of the olive oil and sauté, stirring, for 2–3 minutes over a medium heat. Add the bay leaf, onion and garlic and cook down for another 6 minutes. Add the oregano and both tomato purées/pastes and cook for a further 5 minutes. Add the vegetable stock and simmer for 1 hour uncovered, adding a little water if the pan gets dry.

Once the split peas are tender, turn off the heat and add 2 tablespoons of the remaining olive oil, the vinegar and salt. Remove the bay leaf. Use a hand-held blender to purée the mixture (or process in batches in a tabletop blender). Taste and add black pepper and more salt, if needed. Set aside.

For the griddled cucumber, cut the cucumber into diagonal slices. Brush with the olive oil and season well.

Heat a grill pan/griddle pan until very hot and grill the cucumber slices on both sides until charred. Mix together all the fresh herbs and preserved lemon and use to dress the griddled cucumber.

Fry the reserved sliced cauliflower and sliced olives in the remaining 1 tablespoon oil and then use to garnish the top of the fava. Serve the fava warm or cold with the griddled cucumber on the side and with pitta breads for dipping.

CITRUS CAULI PUDDINGS Ⓥ

Cauliflower makes a perfect undetectable base in this healthy yet delicious dessert. The texture is light and the flavour is sweet and zingy with lemon zest and juice.

SERVES 2

350 g/12 oz. cauliflower, roughly chopped
250 ml/1 cup unsweetened almond milk
1 tablespoon rapadura sugar
1 tablespoon maple syrup
2 teaspoons pure vanilla extract
grated zest and freshly squeezed juice of 2 lemons

TO SERVE

1 white peach, pitted and thinly sliced
handful of blackberries
handful of blueberries
maple syrup, to drizzle
edible flowers (optional)

Add the cauliflower, almond milk, sugar, maple syrup, vanilla extract and lemon zest to a medium pan. Bring to the boil over a medium-high heat, uncovered. Once boiling, reduce the heat to a simmer and cook, uncovered, for about 30 minutes, until the cauliflower is very soft. Remove from the heat.

Add the lemon juice and pour into the bowl of a food processor. Blend on high for 1 minute, or until very smooth. Pour into a clean bowl and allow to cool at room temperature. Cover and refrigerate overnight.

To serve, spoon into two bowls and top with the fruit and a drizzle of maple syrup. Garnish with edible flowers, if you like.

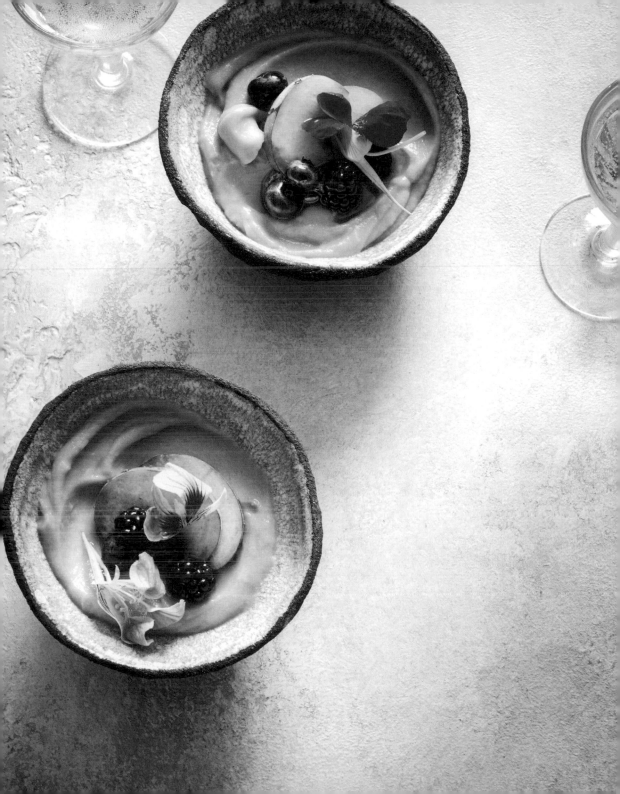

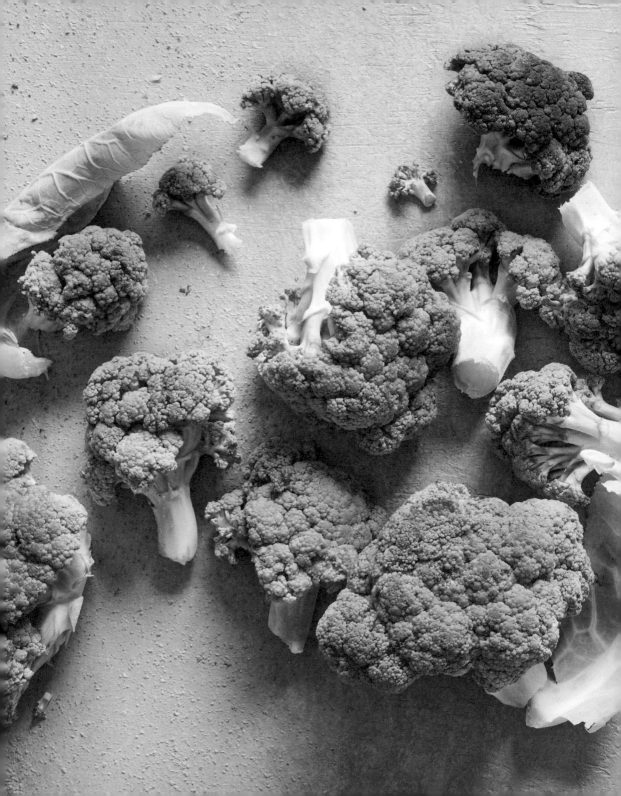

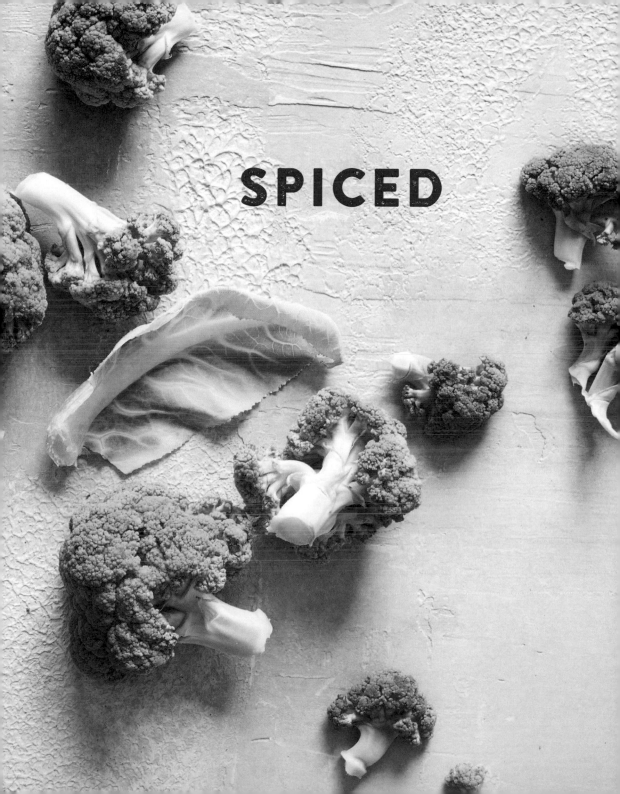

SPICED

CAULIFLOWER LARB WITH COCONUT RICE & FRESH LEAVES Ⓥ

Larb is a flavoursome dish from Northern Thailand that is usually made with meat and served as a salad with rice and crisp leaves. This is my fragrant, sweet and tangy cauliflower version.

SERVES 4

30 g/³/₄ cup coconut chips
3 tablespoons vegetable oil
1 large cauliflower, finely chopped
1 lemongrass stalk, tough outer layers removed, finely chopped
4 fresh kaffir lime leaves, thinly sliced
3 green Thai chillies/chiles, finely chopped
4 tablespoons soy sauce
freshly squeezed juice of 1 lime
5 spring onions/scallions, thinly sliced
10 g/½ cup coriander/cilantro, leaves picked and chopped
10 g/½ cup mint, leaves picked and chopped
salt

TO SERVE
lettuce leaves
cooked jasmine rice
purple basil (optional)

Heat a wok or a large, heavy-based frying pan/skillet over a medium-high heat. Add the coconut chips and cook, stirring, for 2 minutes or until golden brown. Remove from the heat. Transfer to the bowl of a food processor and process until finely ground. Set aside.

Heat the oil in the wok or frying pan/skillet over a high heat. Add the cauliflower, lemongrass, kaffir lime leaves, chillies/chiles, soy sauce and lime juice and cook, stirring occasionally, for 5 minutes or until the cauliflower changes colour. Transfer to a heatproof bowl and set aside for 15 minutes to cool.

Toss the spring onions/scallions, coriander/cilantro and mint into the cauliflower mixture. Season with salt. Serve with lettuce leaves and cooked jasmine rice mixed with the finely ground toasted coconut. Garnish with purple basil, if you like.

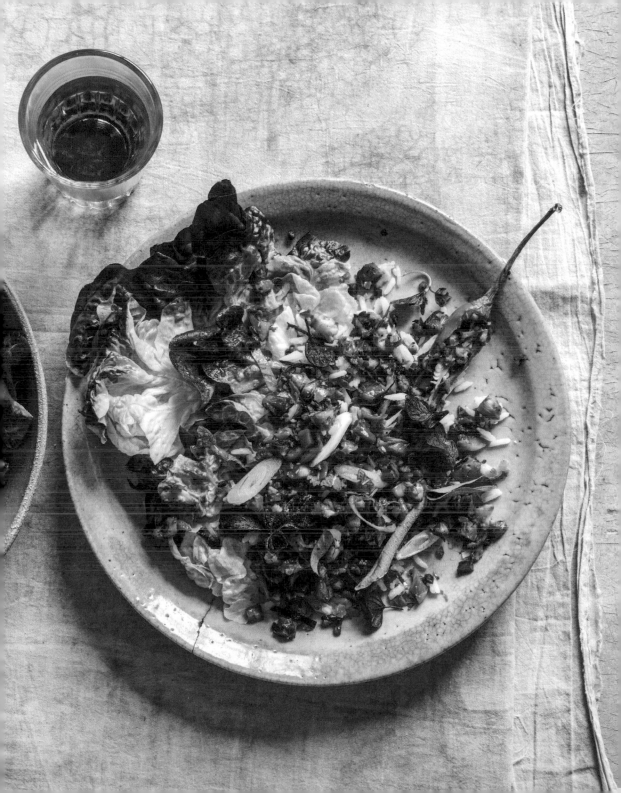

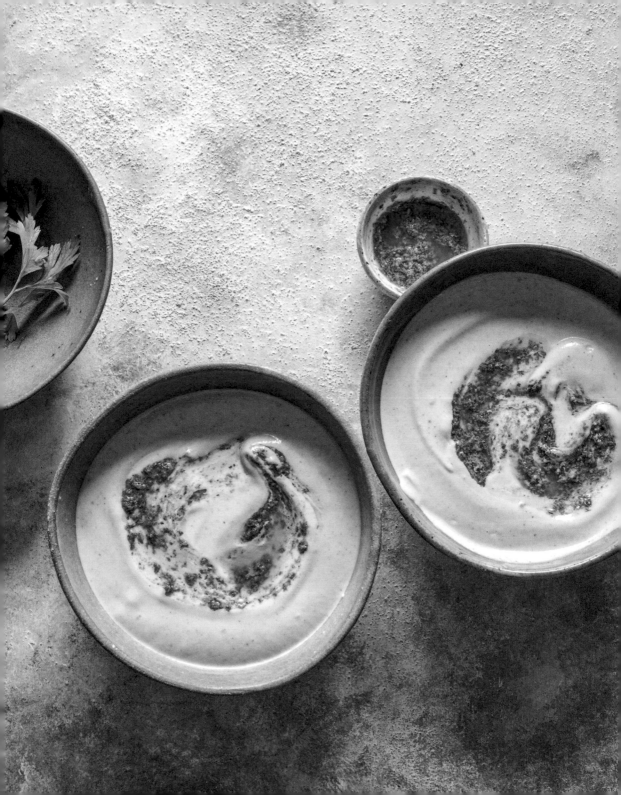

ROAST CAULIFLOWER SOUP WITH ZHOUG

This velvety smooth soup is given a kick with the addition of an earthy spiced herb paste. It's quite hot, so add according to your taste!

SERVES 4–6

SOUP
2 heads of cauliflower, roughly chopped
3 garlic cloves, peeled
2 shallots, roughly chopped
2 tablespoons olive oil
1.5 litres/quarts vegetable stock/broth
4 sprigs thyme, leaves picked
1 bay leaf
150 ml/^{2}/$_3$ cup double/heavy cream
pinch of freshly grated nutmeg
salt and freshly ground black pepper

ZHOUG
50 g/1^3/$_4$ oz. flat-leaf parsley
50 g/1^3/$_4$ oz. coriander/cilantro
8 garlic cloves, peeled
6 bird's eye chillies/chiles, deseeded
seeds from 4–6 crushed cardamom pods
2 tablespoons extra-virgin olive oil, plus extra if needed
^{1}/$_2$ teaspoon salt
^{1}/$_2$ teaspoon freshly ground black pepper

Preheat the oven to 200°C (400°F) Gas 6.

For the soup, in a large baking pan, toss the cauliflower, garlic and shallots with the oil to coat, then roast in the centre of the preheated oven for about 30 minutes, or until golden.

In a large pan, simmer the stock/broth, roasted cauliflower mixture and herbs for 30 minutes, covered, or until the cauliflower is very tender. Discard the bay leaf, then blend the mixture in a blender until smooth. Stir in the cream, nutmeg and some salt and pepper to taste. Heat the soup over a medium heat until just warmed through.

For the zhoug, place the parsley, coriander/cilantro, garlic, chillies/chiles, cardamom seeds, olive oil, salt and pepper in a food processor and process until it forms a spreadable paste (you can add 1 more tablespoon of oil, if needed to make it spreadable).

Serve the soup with the zhoug swirled in, any leftover zhoug can be stored in an airtight container in the fridge for up to a week.

THAI GREEN CAULI CURRY Ⓥ

Aromatic, creamy, fresh and zingy, just like a good Thai curry should be. The addition of liquid aminos in place of the traditional fish sauce adds a depth of flavour and extra umami goodness.

SERVES 4

2 tablespoons coconut oil
2 tablespoons green curry paste
   (check the label says it is vegan,
   if needed)
1 red onion, sliced
4 garlic cloves, crushed
200 g/7 oz. tenderstem cauliflower
   or cauliflower florets
1 red (bell) pepper, deseeded and
   thinly sliced
2 purple or normal carrots, peeled
   and sliced diagonally
2 baby pak choi/bok choy, halved
100 g/3½ oz. mangetout/snow peas
1 tablespoon palm sugar/jaggery
1 tablespoon liquid aminos
   (or tamari)
400-ml/14-fl oz. can coconut milk
3 kaffir lime leaves
freshly squeezed juice of 1 lime
salt and freshly ground black
   pepper

TO SERVE
bunch of purple Thai basil
sambal oelek (optional)
cooked rice
lime wedges

In a large pan or wok set over a medium-high heat, heat 1 tablespoon of the coconut oil, being cautious of it spitting.

Add the curry paste and fry it, stirring it into the coconut oil, for about 1 minute. Turn the heat down, add the onion and cook until the onion is slightly translucent, about 8 minutes.

Add the garlic, stir together, then add the second tablespoon of coconut oil. Add the cauliflower, red (bell) pepper, carrots, pak choi/bok choy and mangetout/snow peas. Add the palm sugar/jaggery, liquid aminos (or tamari) and some salt and pepper and stir everything together. Reduce the heat to medium and cook down, stirring, until the carrots are tender-crisp, about 10–15 minutes.

Add the coconut milk and kaffir lime leaves, stir, and then let it simmer for about 5 minutes. Squeeze the lime juice over, stir, and then remove from the heat.

Add the purple Thai basil and stir in the sambal oelek, if using. Serve with rice and lime wedges.

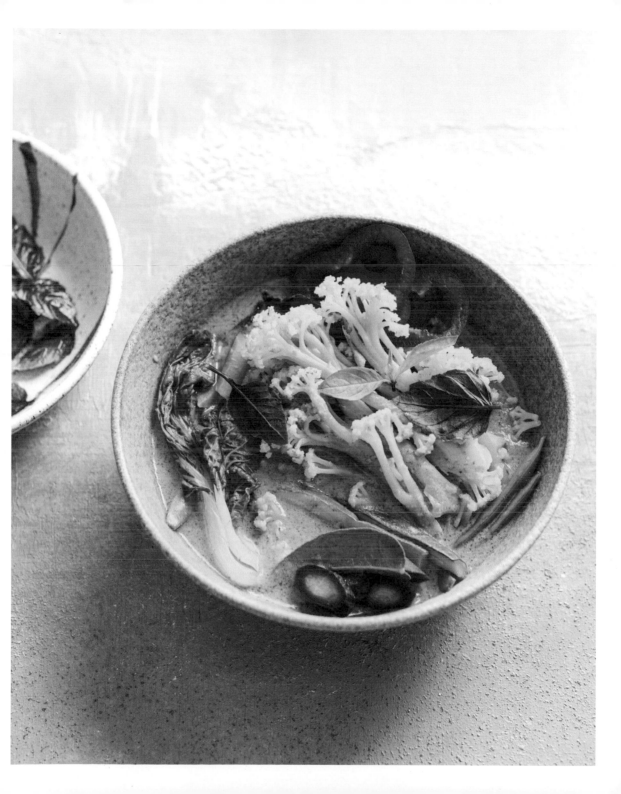

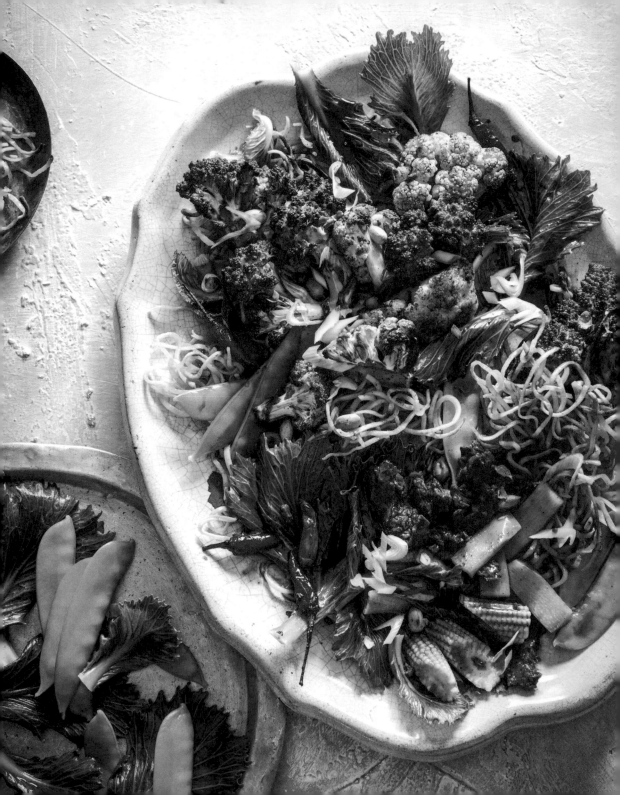

FIVE-SPICE CAULI BAKE
WITH CRISPY NOODLES & TOFU

A fusion of crispy noodles, vegetables, spice-roasted cauliflower and
seitan in an Asian sauce. Pile it all on a platter and let everyone dig in!

SERVES 4

½ head each of Romanesco broccoli
   and cauliflower, cut into florets
2 tablespoons runny honey
1 tablespoon five spice powder
2 tablespoons soy sauce
6 garlic cloves, peeled
5–6 red Thai chillies/chiles
salt and freshly ground black pepper

CRISPY NOODLES
225 g/8 oz. fresh thin egg noodles
2 tablespoons groundnut oil

SEITAN IN SAUCE
200 g/7 oz. seitan pieces
5-cm/2-inch piece of ginger, grated
6 tablespoons Shaoxing rice wine
4 tablespoons vegetarian oyster
   sauce
2 tablespoons light soy sauce

TO FINISH
100 g/3½ oz. mangetout/snow
   peas, blanched and refreshed
100 g/3½ oz. baby corn, blanched
   and refreshed
100 g/3½ oz. kale, blanched and
   refreshed
120 g/4 oz. canned bamboo shoots
50 g/generous ⅓ cup peanuts,
   roasted and chopped
6 spring onions/scallions, chopped

Preheat the oven to 200°C (400°F) Gas 6.

Place the Romanesco broccoli and cauliflower on a lined
baking sheet. In a small bowl, stir together the honey,
five-spice, soy sauce and some salt and pepper until well
combined. Drizzle over the vegetables, then add the garlic
and chillies/chiles. Roast in the preheated oven for 10
minutes, then take them out and give a light stir to ensure
even browning, and roast again for another 5–10 minutes
until they are browned all over. Remove from the oven and
let them cool slightly on the baking sheet.

For the crispy noodles, place a large frying pan/skillet
over a medium-high heat. Add the noodles and oil and allow
to crisp up before turning. Repeat for 10–15 minutes. There
should be a combination of crispy edges and soft noodles.

For the seitan in sauce, place a saucepan over a medium-
high heat. Add all the ingredients with seasoning and bring
to the boil. Cook for 5 minutes, then remove from the heat.

To serve, place the crispy noodles, the roasted vegetables
and the seitan in sauce on a platter and finish with the
mangetout/snow peas, baby corn, kale and bamboo shoots.
Serve scattered with the chopped roasted peanuts and
spring onions/scallions.

CAULIFLOWER KATSU CURRY

The katsu is a Japanese curry and is generally thicker, milder and sweeter than an Indian curry. It is traditionally served with chicken but is absolutely delicious served with a breaded cauliflower steak.

SERVES 2

5 tablespoons plain/
   all-purpose flour
1 cauliflower, cut into
   rounds (steaks)
100 g/2⅓ cups panko breadcrumbs
2 tablespoons flavourless oil, plus
   extra as needed
1 onion, thinly sliced
2 garlic cloves, finely chopped
5-cm/2-inch piece of fresh ginger,
   finely grated
1 tablespoon curry powder
600 ml/2½ cups vegetable stock
2 tablespoons soy sauce
2 teaspoons runny honey
2 teaspoons rice vinegar
1 teaspoon garam masala
2–3 tablespoons coconut cream
salt and freshly ground black pepper
boiled rice, to serve
micro herbs, to garnish (optional)

QUICK PICKLE

1 carrot, peeled and julienned
1–2 mini courgettes/zucchini, thinly
   sliced diagonally
4 radishes, trimmed and sliced
2 tablespoons rice vinegar
1 teaspoon caster/granulated sugar
2 teaspoons sesame seeds
pinch of salt

In a large bowl, combine 3 tablespoons of the flour with enough water to make a runny paste, then season and add the cauliflower rounds, tossing until they are all coated. Tip the breadcrumbs onto a plate and dip in each cauliflower round, pressing down to help the crumbs stick all over.

Preheat the oven to 180°C (350°F) Gas 4.

Heat the oil in a frying pan/skillet. Cook the cauliflower in batches for 5 minutes on each side, adding a little more oil between batches if needed. Transfer the slices to a baking sheet as you go. Once all the cauliflower is browned, place the baking sheet in the preheated oven and cook for 10–15 minutes while you make the sauce.

Meanwhile, make the quick pickle. Combine all the ingredients in a bowl with a pinch of salt, and set aside.

Wipe out the frying pan/skillet and heat another drizzle of oil. Add the onion and cook for a few minutes to soften. Stir in the garlic, ginger and curry powder for 1 minute, then add the remaining 2 tablespoons flour. Gently add the stock, little by little, stirring for a smooth sauce. Add the soy sauce, honey, rice vinegar, garam masala and coconut cream, then simmer over a low heat for 10 minutes, adding a splash of water if it gets too thick.

Serve the crispy cauliflower steaks and sauce with boiled rice and the quick pickle on the side. Garnish with micro herbs, if you like.

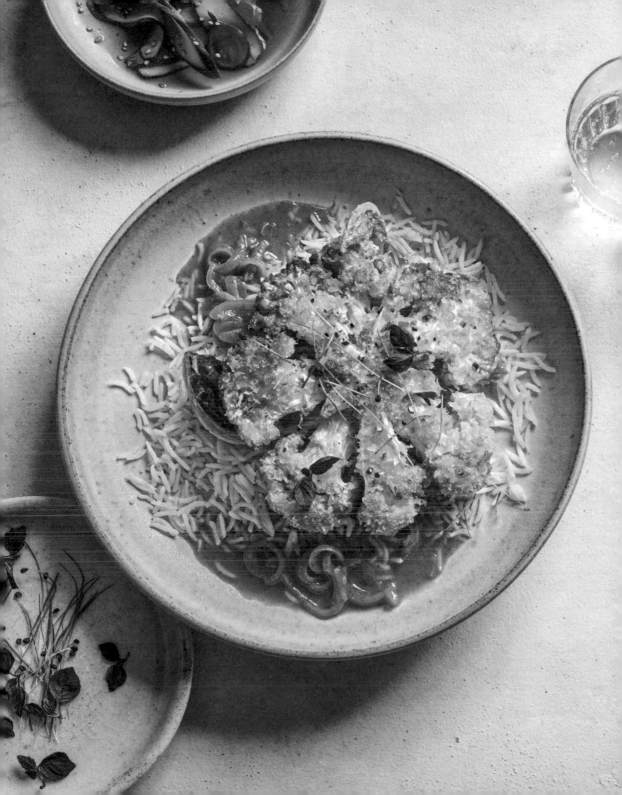

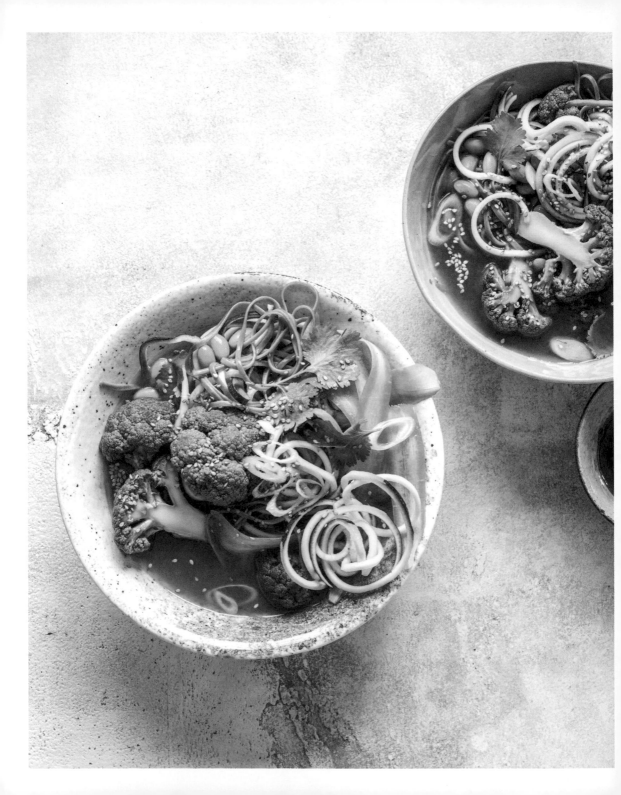

DAN DAN CAULIFLOWER SOUP Ⓥ

This Dan Dan Noodle Soup is a flavour explosion in a bowl. It is also
a very healthy meal which you can have on the table in no time at all.
Use whatever accompanying vegetables are in season.

SERVES 4

400 g/14 oz. rice noodles
300 g/10½ oz. caulifower, cut
    into florets
1 carrot, peeled and thinly sliced
    diagonally with a peeler
2 courgettes/zucchini, spiralized
100 g/¾ cup frozen edamame
    beans

STOCK
1 litre/quart good-quality vegetable
    stock
3 garlic cloves, crushed
4-cm/1½-inch piece of fresh
    ginger, grated
3 teaspoons palm sugar/jaggery

STOCK SAUCE
3 tablespoons light soy sauce
2 tablespoons tahini
4 tablespoons black vinegar
    (not balsamic)
2 teaspoons dark soy sauce
1 teaspoon kecap manis
1 teaspoon chilli/chili oil, plus extra
    to garnish
2 teaspoons sesame oil

TO GARNISH
spring onions/scallions, sliced
coriander/cilantro, leaves picked
toasted sesame seeds

Combine all the stock ingredients in a large saucepan and
bring to the boil. Meanwhile, mix the stock sauce ingredients
together in a small bowl.

When the stock comes to the boil, place the rice noodles
in the stock, then 1 minute later, add the cauliflower and
carrot. After another 1 minute, remove the pot from the
heat and add the rest of the veg and the stock sauce. Mix
well, taste and adjust the seasoning, if required, with extra
splashes of ingredients from the stock sauce.

Divide the noodles and vegetables between four bowls.
Ladle the soup into the bowls over the vegetables and
noodles, and garnish with some sliced spring onions/
scallions, coriander/cilantro leaves and toasted sesame seeds
– plus some extra chilli/chili oil if you can handle the heat!

LAKSA WITH CAULIFLOWER Ⓥ

Laksa, the epic Malaysian spicy coconut noodle soup, is a must-try at least once in your life! The soup is rich, fragrant, a bit spicy and loaded with lots of vegetables.

SERVES 4

CRISPY TOFU
200 g/7 oz. firm tofu, drained
1 tablespoon cornflour/cornstarch
salt
2 tablespoons vegetable oil,
    for frying

LAKSA
1 tablespoon vegetable oil
4 tablespoons vegan laksa paste
1 litre/quart vegetable stock
1 tablespoon soy sauce
1 tablespoon palm sugar/jaggery
400-ml/14-fl oz. can coconut milk
200 g/7 oz. cauliflower, cut into
    florets or mini cauliflowers
80 g/3 oz. mini courgettes/zucchini
100 g/3½ oz. asparagus tips
freshly squeezed juice of 1–2 limes
200 g/7 oz. rice/soba noodles

TO FINISH
50 g/scant 1 cup beansprouts
3 spring onions/scallions, sliced
    diagonally
10 g/½ cup coriander/cilantro,
    leaves picked
1 red chilli/chile, sliced diagonally
lime wedges
chilli/chili sauce

For the crispy tofu, line a plate with a folded paper towel and set the tofu on top. Set a small plate on top of the tofu and weigh it down with something heavy. Pat the tofu dry with more towels. Cut into cubes, season with salt and evenly coat with the cornflour/cornstarch. Heat the oil in a frying pan/skillet and add all of the tofu in a single layer. The tofu should sizzle upon contact – if not, wait a few minutes to let the pan heat up more. At first, the tofu will stick to the pan, so wait until the tofu releases from the pan before browning the next side. Fry until all sides are brown and crispy. Transfer to a cooling rack. It will remain crisp only for a few hours.

For the laksa, heat a wok over a high heat and add the oil. Swirl to coat. Add the laksa paste and cook, stirring, for 3 minutes or until fragrant. Add the stock, soy sauce and palm sugar/jaggery, and bring to the boil. Reduce the heat to medium. Add the coconut milk and simmer for 5 minutes. Add the cauliflower, mini courgettes/zucchini and asparagus tips, and cook for 2 minutes. Remove from the heat and add the lime juice to taste. Stir to combine.

Meanwhile, place the noodles in a heatproof bowl. Cover with boiling water and leave to stand for 5 minutes or until tender. Drain and divide the noodles between four bowls. Ladle the coconut mixture over the noodles. Serve with the crispy tofu, beansprouts, spring onions/scallions, coriander/cilantro, chilli/chile and lime wedges, and an extra drizzle of chilli/chili sauce.

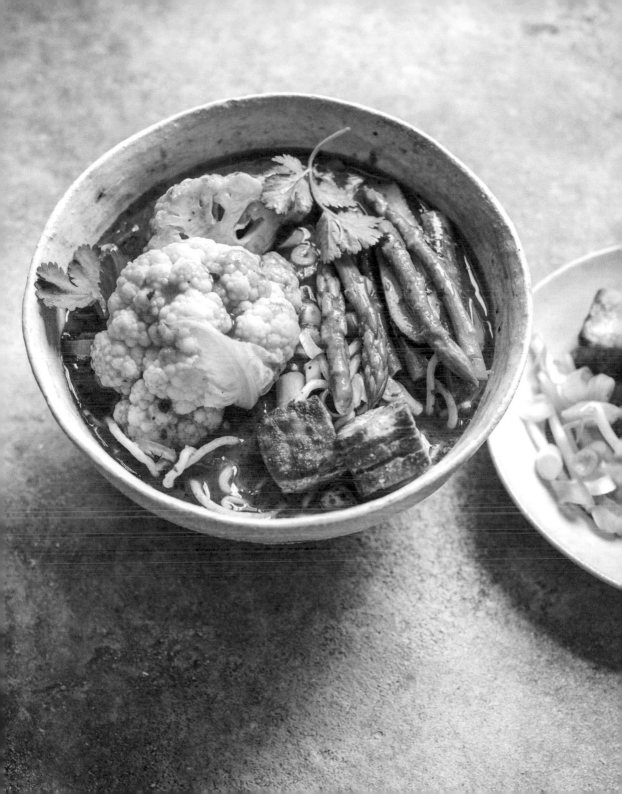

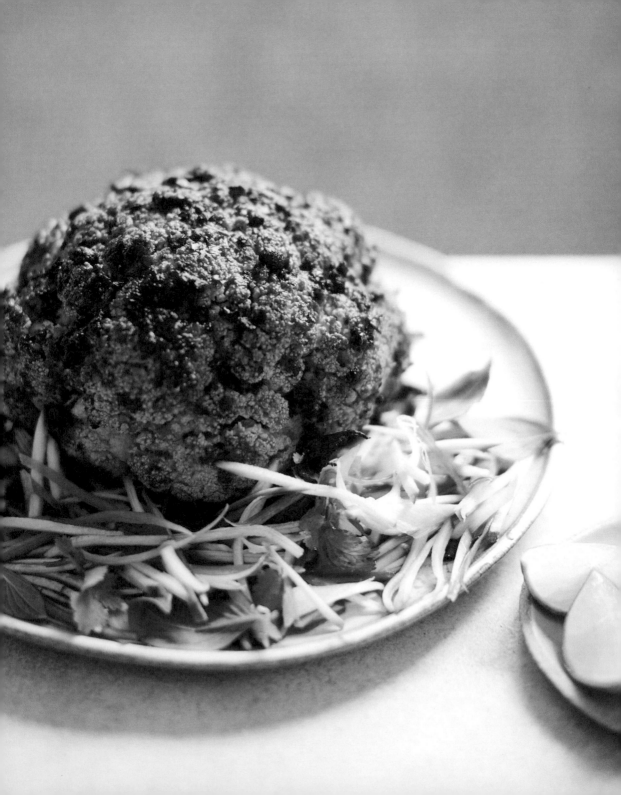

MISO & BLACK BEAN CHILLI WHOLE-BAKED CAULIFLOWER WITH SESAME NOODLES

A great mid-week meal, this recipe is inspired by my lovely friend, Rosie Reynolds. The combination of miso with black bean chilli sauce is a delicious mix and goes perfectly with cauliflower.

SERVES 4 AS AN APPETIZER

1 whole cauliflower, stalk trimmed
3 tablespoons sake
3 tablespoons mirin
100 g/3½ oz. miso paste
1 tablespoon soft brown sugar
50 g/1¾ oz. black bean chilli/chili sauce
3 teaspoons sesame oil
salt

SESAME NOODLES

200 g/7 oz. buckwheat noodles
1 tablespoon tahini
1 tablespoon peanut butter
1–2 tablespoons light soy sauce
1 tablespoon rice vinegar
1 tablespoon vegetable oil
1 tablespoon maple syrup
4 spring onions/scallions, sliced diagonally

TO SERVE

1 courgette/zucchini, shredded
1 carrot, peeled and shredded
lime wedges
handful of Thai basil
handful of coriander/cilantro

Preheat the oven to 200°C (400°F) Gas 6.

Bring a pot three-quarters full of salted water and large enough to fit the cauliflower in to the boil. Add the cauliflower and cook for 5–10 minutes or until a skewer goes in easily. Remove carefully and place in a small roasting pan.

While the cauliflower is cooking, combine the sake and mirin in a small saucepan over a medium heat. Whisk in the miso paste and then stir in the sugar until dissolved. Remove from the heat and stir in the black bean chilli/chili sauce and sesame oil. Pour the black bean miso glaze over the cauliflower and roast in the preheated oven for 30 minutes, basting occasionally. Cover with foil if it gets too dark. Keep warm until ready to serve.

Meanwhile, cook the noodles according to the package instructions. While the noodles are cooking, make the sauce by mixing together the tahini, peanut butter, light soy sauce, rice vinegar, vegetable oil, maple syrup and 2 tablespoons of water. Stir to a smooth, even paste.

Once the noodles are cooked, drain them and toss with the prepared sauce and spring onions/scallions. It's best to mix the noodles while they are still hot.

Serve the cauliflower on a bed of the courgette/zucchini and carrot, with the sesame noodles and lime wedges on the side. Garnish with Thai basil and coriander/cilantro.

CAULIFLOWER TANDOOR

This all-in-one tandoor-style dish is perfect to share with friends.
Serve pickles, chutneys and breads on the side for a full Indian feast.
For a vegan take, omit the paneer and use a plant-based yogurt.

SERVES 4

450 g/1 lb. new potatoes, scrubbed
4 garlic cloves, peeled
5-cm/2-inch piece of fresh ginger,
    grated
3 tablespoons tandoori spice blend
freshly squeezed juice of 1 lemon
1 teaspoon salt
160 ml/²/₃ cup coconut cream
1 large head of cauliflower, leaves
    removed and halved
2 long green chillies/chiles, halved
    lengthways
150 g/5¹/₂ oz. cherry tomatoes
200 g/7 oz. paneer, cut into cubes
200 g/7 oz. kale, blanched
papadums, to serve
lime wedges, to serve

MINT YOGURT
150 g/5¹/₂ oz. natural/plain yogurt
10 g/¹/₂ cup mint, leaves picked and
    chopped
grated zest and freshly squeezed
    juice of ¹/₂ lime
salt and freshly ground black
    pepper

Start by boiling the potatoes in a pan of salted water for 20 minutes until tender. Drain and place into a baking dish.

Preheat the oven to 180°C (350°F) Gas 4.

In a food processor, blitz the garlic and ginger into a paste. Add the tandoori spice, lemon juice and salt and mix until uniform. Fold in 120 ml/¹/₂ cup of the coconut cream. Place the cauliflower in a large bowl and spread the marinade all over, making sure to coat the bottom as well.

In the same baking dish as the potatoes, place the cauliflower and the halved chillies/chiles, then roast in the preheated oven covered with foil until tender, about 45–60 minutes, depending on the size of the cauliflower. For the last 10 minutes of cooking, remove the foil, increase the oven temperature to 190°C (375°F) Gas 5 and add the cherry tomatoes, the cubed paneer and the remaining coconut cream. Remove from the oven. While the dish is still hot, add the blanched kale and allow it to wilt in the heat.

Mix the mint yogurt ingredients together in a small bowl, and serve the roasted cauliflower mixture with papadums, the mint yogurt and some lime wedges.

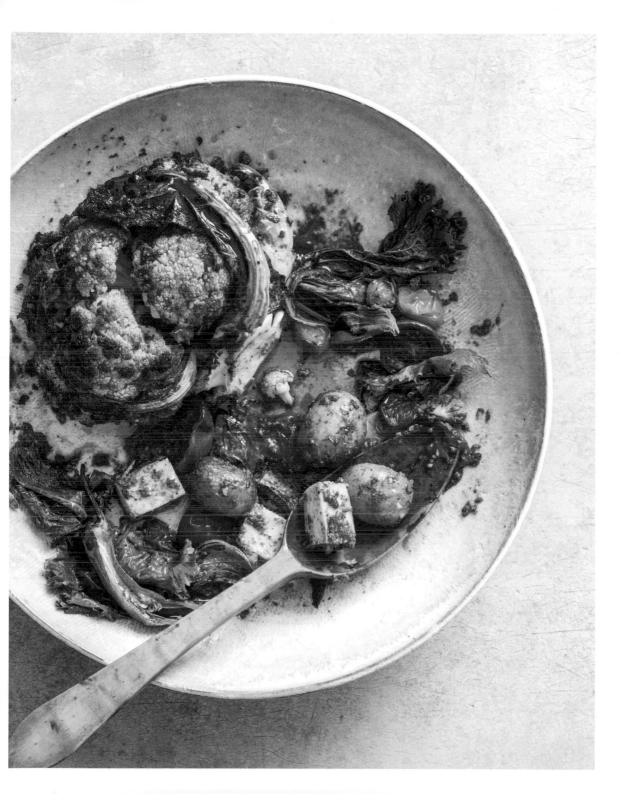

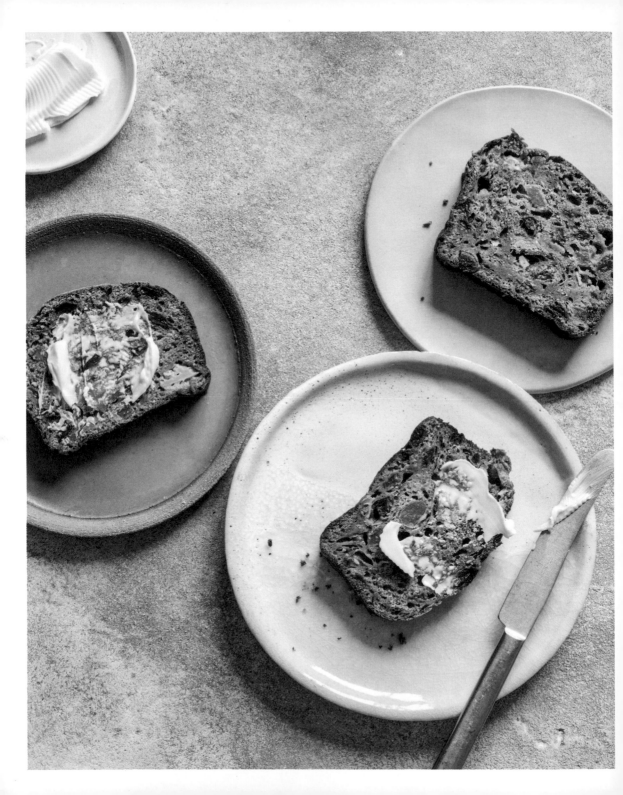

CAULIFLOWER COURGETTE SPICE LOAF

This is best served on the day it is made, still a little warm from the oven, spread with butter. The next day, toast it, drizzle with maple syrup and serve with yogurt.

MAKES 1 FAMILY-SIZED TEA LOAF

40 g/3 tablespoons unsalted butter

70 g/2¹/₂ oz. courgette/zucchini, coarsely grated

120 g/4 oz. cauliflower, blitzed in a food processor

100 g/³/₄ cup sultanas/golden raisins

50 g/¹/₃ cup dried apricots, chopped

125 ml/¹/₂ cup full-fat natural/plain yogurt

2 UK large/US extra-large eggs

75 g/6 tablespoons caster/superfine sugar

1 teaspoon ground cinnamon

¹/₂ teaspoon ground ginger

¹/₂ teaspoon ground cloves

¹/₂ teaspoon ground cardamom

75 g/¹/₂ cup wholemeal/whole-wheat flour

200 g/1¹/₂ cups plain/all-purpose flour

2¹/₂ teaspoons baking powder

¹/₄ teaspoon salt

900-g/2-lb loaf pan, lined

Preheat the oven to 170°C (325°F) Gas 3.

Melt the butter in a pan over a low heat, then set aside to cool slightly while you prepare the remaining ingredients.

Combine the courgette/zucchini, cauliflower, sultanas/golden raisins, dried apricots, yogurt, eggs, sugar and spices in a mixing bowl. Stir in the melted butter. In a separate bowl, combine the flours, baking powder and salt. Add these dry ingredients to the wet mixture in the mixing bowl, and stir lightly until just combined.

Spoon the mixture into the prepared loaf pan and level the top. Bake in the preheated oven for 60–65 minutes or until a small knife inserted into the middle comes out clean. Let cool a little, then turn out of the pan and leave to cool completely. Cut into slices to serve, toasted if you like, and spread with plenty of butter.

INDIAN-SPICED CAULI BURGERS

These open cauli burgers served on naan bread make a great alternative to a classic burger. You can freeze some of the burgers for another time if needed.

MAKES 10

200 g/7 oz. quinoa
1 head of cauliflower
3–4 tablespoons olive oil
1 teaspoon ground cumin
1 teaspoon ground coriander
1 teaspoon chilli/chili powder
  (optional)
2 garlic cloves, crushed
100 g/1¼ cups dried breadcrumbs
50 g/½ cup ground almonds
100 g/1 cup grated paneer
3 eggs
2 green chillies/chiles, finely
  chopped
handful of coriander/cilantro,
  finely chopped
salt and freshly ground black
  pepper

TO SERVE

small round naan breads
raita
mango chutney
spring onions/scallions, thinly sliced
lettuce leaves
coriander/cilantro
shaved cucumber ribbons
lime wedges, for squeezing

baking sheet, lined

Preheat the oven to 200°C (400°F) Gas 6.

Cook the quinoa according to the package instructions. Drain, leave to cool in the sieve/strainer and pat dry with paper towels to remove as much moisture as possible.

Cut the cauliflower into florets, transfer to a baking sheet, drizzle with 1 tablespoon of the oil and sprinkle with the spices to taste. Roast in the preheated oven for 20–30 minutes, then leave to cool. Pulse in a food processor to roughly chop into small pieces that stick together.

Combine the cooked, pulsed cauliflower with the quinoa, garlic, breadcrumbs, ground almonds, paneer, eggs, green chillies/chiles, coriander/cilantro and some salt and pepper.

Divide the mixture into 10 portions, then shape each one into a small patty/burger.

Place the burgers on the lined baking sheet and bake in the preheated oven for 25–30 minutes until golden. Serve each burger on a naan bread, with some raita, mango chutney, spring onions/scallions, lettuce leaves, coriander/cilantro, shaved cucumber ribbons and a squeeze of lime.

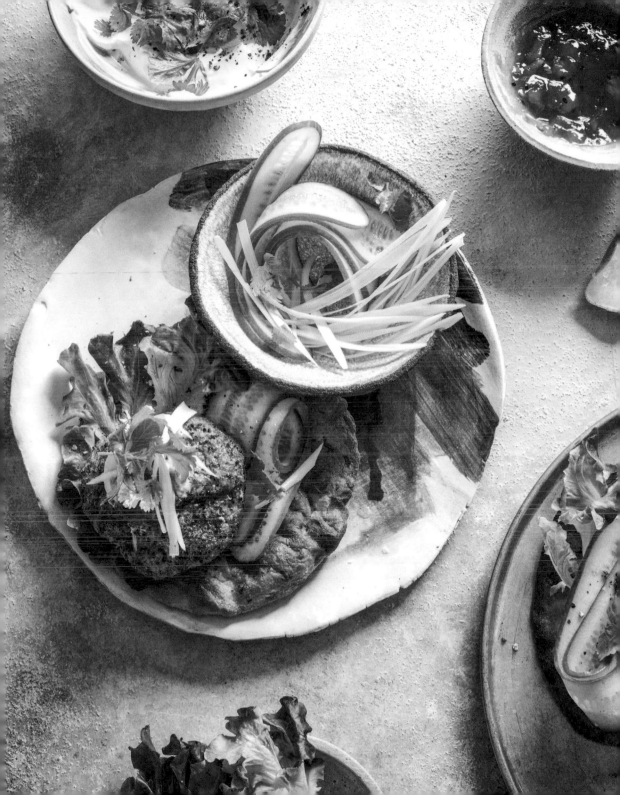

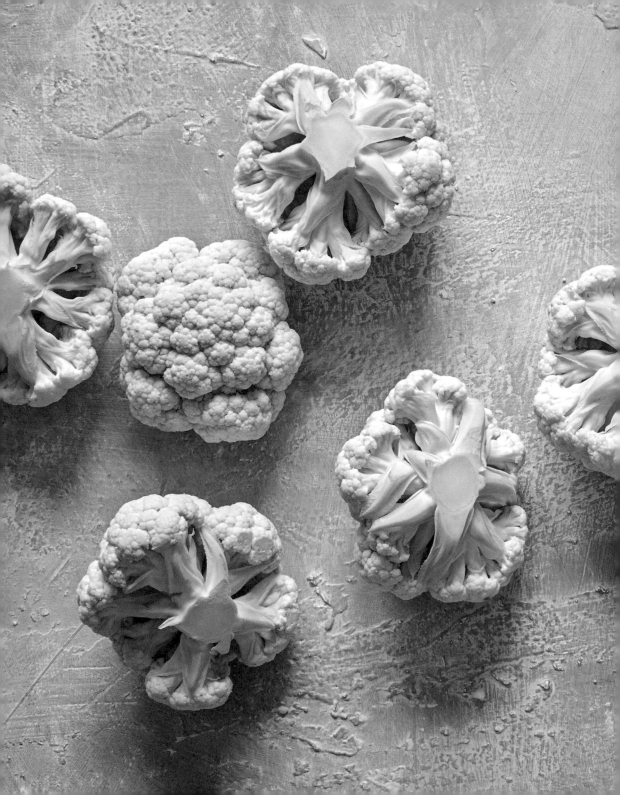

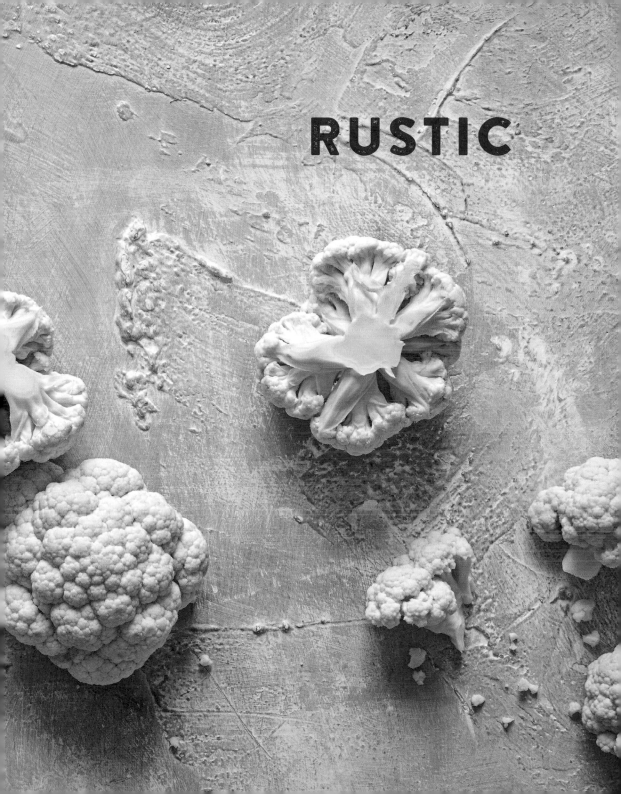

RUSTIC

CAULIFLOWER PUTTANESCA PIZZA

A combination of punchy ingredients – capers, black olives and chillies/chiles – along with creamy mozzarella and fresh basil, accompany this gluten-free and low-carb cauliflower pizza base.

SERVES 2

500 g/1 lb. 2 oz. cauliflower florets
2 eggs, beaten
100 g/1 cup ground almonds
3 sprigs thyme, leaves picked
2 garlic cloves, crushed
½ teaspoon dried chilli flakes/hot red pepper flakes
2 tablespoons olive oil
150 ml/⅔ cup passata/strained tomatoes
1 tablespoon capers, drained
1 tablespoon pitted black olives, chopped
1 ball of mozzarella, torn
salt and freshly ground black pepper
basil leaves, to serve

baking sheet, lined and sprayed with oil

Preheat the oven to 200°C (400°F) Gas 6.

Cook the cauliflower in boiling salted water for 4 minutes, then drain well. Once cooled, pat with a kitchen towel to dry it completely and transfer to a food processor. Blitz until it resembles couscous. Tip into a bowl, season, and stir in the eggs, ground almonds and thyme. Mix until it comes together. Spread onto the lined baking sheet and press into a pizza base-shape using a spatula. Bake in the preheated oven for 15–20 minutes until it is golden and firm.

Meanwhile, in a frying pan/skillet, fry the garlic and chilli flakes/hot red pepper flakes in the olive oil for a minute before adding the passata/strained tomatoes. Simmer and reduce for 30 minutes, until thick and spreadable, then season. Add the capers and olives.

Spread the tomato sauce over the pizza base, then add the mozzarella. Return to the oven for 10–12 minutes until the cheese has turned golden. Scatter with basil and serve.

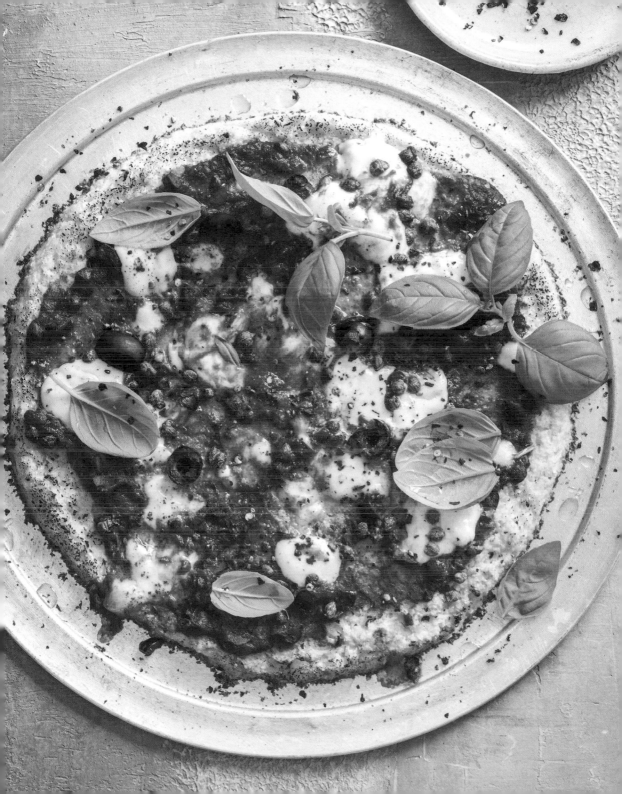

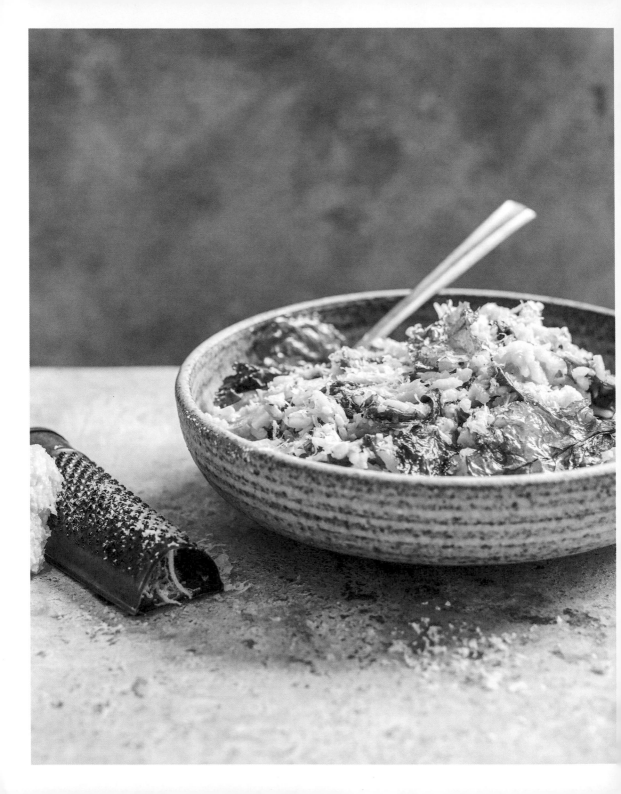

CAULIFLOWER RISOTTO

This risotto is made with half cauli 'rice' and half risotto rice. It has the creaminess of a traditional risotto, but the cauliflower gives it more nutritious value and is lower in carbohydrates.

SERVES 4

20 g/1½ tablespoons unsalted butter
drizzle of olive oil
1 onion, finely chopped
250 g/1⅓ cups risotto rice
big pinch of saffron threads
90 ml/⅓ cup dry white wine
900 ml–1 litre/scant 4 cups–1 quart hot vegetable stock
40 g/1½ oz. Parmesan cheese (or vegetarian hard cheese alternative), finely grated, plus extra to serve
grated zest and freshly squeezed juice of 1 lemon
1 head of cauliflower (400 g/14 oz.), grated or blitzed in a food processor
100 g/2 cups baby kale leaves

Melt the butter in a large saucepan set over a low heat with a drizzle of olive oil. Add the onion and cook for 10–15 minutes, until soft but not coloured.

Turn the heat up to medium, then pour in the risotto rice and stir for a few minutes, to ensure every grain is well coated in butter, then add the saffron and stir well.

Pour in the white wine and let it bubble away for a couple of minutes, stirring regularly.

Begin ladling in the hot vegetable stock, bit by bit, stirring it through the rice and allowing each ladleful to become absorbed before adding the next. Continue slowly adding stock in this way for about 15–20 minutes until the rice is cooked through and the risotto is creamy.

Stir in the grated cheese, lemon zest and juice, grated cauliflower and baby kale and cook for a further 3 minutes. Serve with extra grated cheese on top.

CAULIFLOWER & POTATO HASH WITH EGGS

Why should hashes be reserved for brunch? I could eat this at any time. It would also be perfect served on a bed of salad instead of eggs.

SERVES 2

3 baby potatoes, scrubbed
   and chopped
1 sweet potato, scrubbed and
   roughly chopped
1 tablespoon olive oil, plus extra
   for frying the eggs
1 tablespoon ghee
1 red onion, finely chopped
300 g/10$\frac{1}{2}$ oz. chopped cauliflower
   (use a mix of florets and stems)
200 g/7 oz. cherry tomatoes, halved
3 garlic cloves, smashed
30 g/1 cup coarsely chopped
   flat-leaf parsley
2 eggs
salt and freshly ground black
   pepper
handful of mixed soft herbs, such
   as parsley, coriander/cilantro,
   dill or mint, to serve
Sriracha, to serve (optional)

Place the chopped baby potatoes and sweet potato in a small saucepan of salted water and bring to the boil. After 5 minutes at a rolling boil, drain and set aside.

Heat the olive oil and ghee in a frying pan/skillet, then add the red onion, cauliflower and boiled potatoes and cook over a medium-high heat for about 7–9 minutes, stirring occasionally.

Add the tomatoes, garlic and parsley and cook for 5–10 minutes or until the cauliflower and potatoes are browned and the tomatoes start to blister. Keep turning until everything is brown and the edges are crisped up, and the tomatoes are caramelized.

Meanwhile, in another frying pan/skillet, fry the eggs in a little oil and then serve with the hash. Season well with salt and pepper and finish with herbs and Sriracha, if you like.

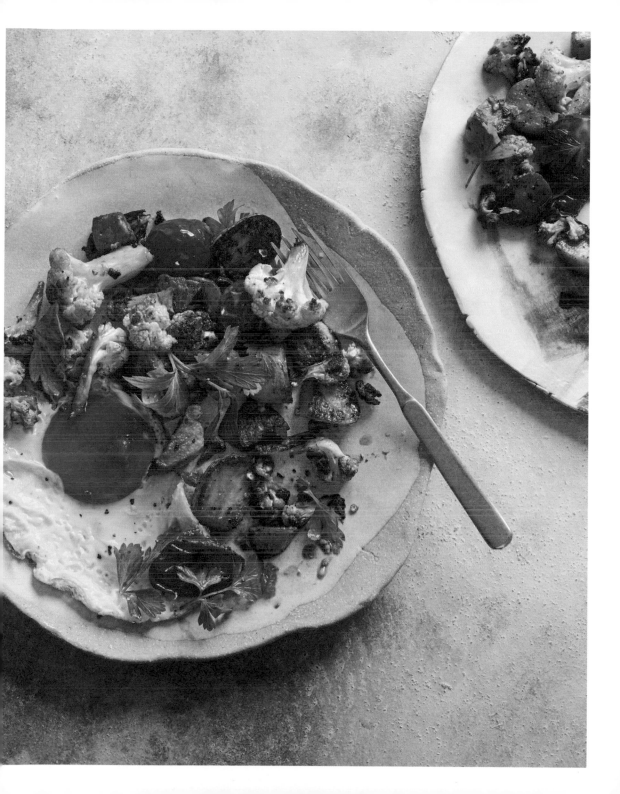

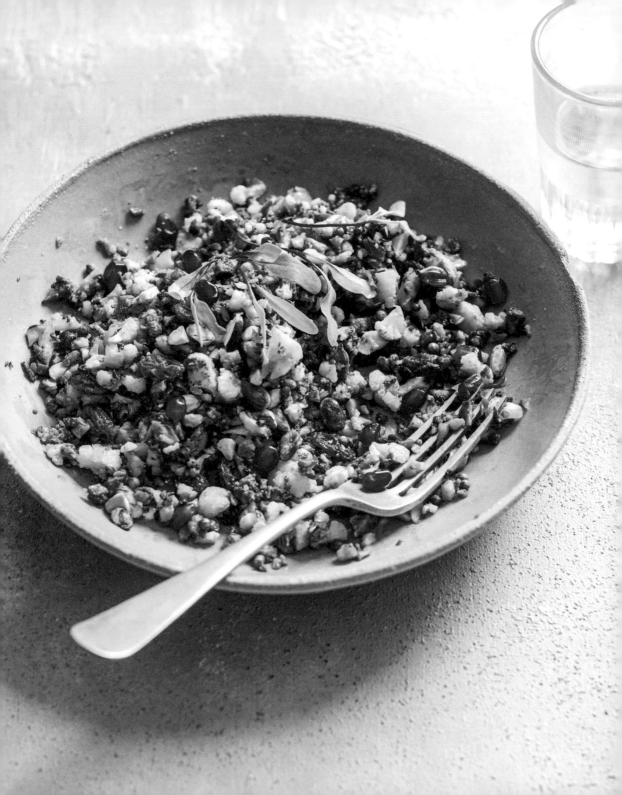

QUICK CAULIFLOWER RICE SAFFRON PILAF Ⓥ

This is the perfect low-carb side dish, and you can really have fun with it by adding extra herbs or spices to taste. For a quick, healthy meal, I serve this with lots of steamed green vegetables and some chilli sauce.

SERVES 2

50 ml/3½ tablespoons coconut cream
large pinch of saffron threads
1 medium head of cauliflower
1 tablespoon coconut oil
1 onion, finely chopped
1 tablespoon pomegranate seeds
1 tablespoon pistachios
salt and freshly ground black pepper
micro herbs, to garnish (optional)

Warm the coconut cream through in a small saucepan over a low heat. Turn off the heat, then add the saffron threads and leave to steep.

Meanwhile, remove the core from the cauliflower and cut it into florets, leaving some stem on each. In 2–3 batches, add the cauliflower florets to a food processor with the blade attachment and pulse a few times until the cauliflower is processed into rice-sized pieces. Set aside.

Add the coconut oil to a medium sauté pan or frying pan/skillet over a medium heat. When the oil is hot, add the onion and sauté for about 3–4 minutes or until translucent.

Add the cauliflower 'rice' and sauté for 10 minutes until slightly browned. Turn the heat down to low, then stir in the coconut saffron mixture and allow to absorb for a few minutes.

Finally, stir through the pomegranate seeds and pistachios and season with salt and pepper. Serve garnished with micro herbs, if you like.

SIMPLE RUSTIC SALAD Ⓥ

This is inspired by a gorgeous roasted salad they serve at the
Divertimenti café in London. I honestly make this simplified version
at least once a week and probably for every barbecue or cookout.

SERVES 4

1 head of cauliflower, cut into
   wedges
5 garlic cloves, crushed into a paste
½ bunch fresh thyme, leaves picked
3 tablespoons olive oil
pinch of dried chilli flakes/hot red
   pepper flakes
60 g/2¼ oz. capers, rinsed and
   drained
100 g/3½ oz. semi-dried tomatoes
200 g/7 oz. torn sourdough
20 g/1 cup (loosely packed) fresh
   parsley, leaves picked and roughly
   chopped
1 tablespoon balsamic reduction,
   to finish

Preheat the oven to 200°C (400°F) Gas 6.

Place the cauliflower in a large baking dish and rub
with the crushed garlic, thyme and olive oil. Roast in the
preheated oven for 30 minutes.

Remove from the oven and sprinkle with the dried chilli
flakes/hot red pepper flakes, capers, semi-dried tomatoes
and torn sourdough. Return to the oven for another
20 minutes until the cauliflower is nicely browned.

Serve scattered with the chopped parsley and drizzled
with the balsamic reduction.

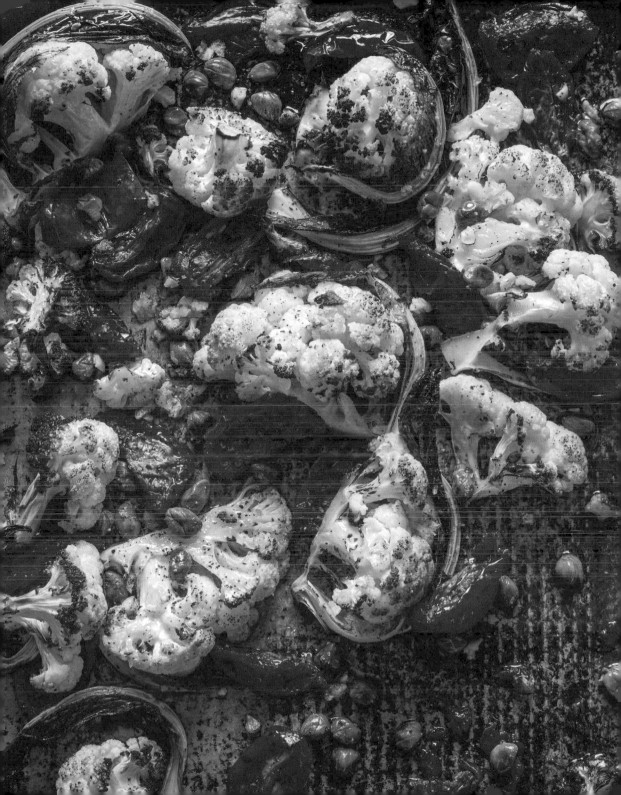

CAULI SAMOSAS

Ideal for entertaining, serve these flavourful little samosas as party finger food or to accompany an Indian feast.

MAKES 18–20 DEPENDING ON SIZE

1 red chilli/chile
2 garlic cloves, roughly chopped
3-cm/1¼-inch piece of fresh ginger, peeled and
  roughly chopped
175 g/6 oz. potatoes, unpeeled
200 g/7 oz. cauliflower, cut into small florets
50 ml/3½ tablespoons vegetable oil
1 onion, finely chopped
½ teaspoon asafoetida
1 teaspoon black mustard seeds
2 teaspoon cumin seeds
80 g/scant ⅔ cup frozen peas
1 tablespoon ground coriander
2 teaspoon garam masala
1 tablespoon freshly chopped coriander/cilantro
18–20 spring roll wrappers
salt and freshly ground black pepper
500 ml/2 cups vegetable oil, for deep-frying

Blitz the chilli/chile, garlic and ginger in a blender to make a fairly smooth paste.

Boil the potatoes for 15 minutes. While they are boiling, place the cauliflower florets on top to steam for the last 3 minutes. Drain the potatoes and, when cool, remove the skins and chop roughly intro 1-cm/½-inch cubes.

Heat the oil in a large pan over a medium heat and, when hot, add the onion, asafoetida, black mustard seeds and cumin seeds and fry for 1 minute. Add the potatoes, cauliflower, peas, ground coriander and salt and pepper, as well as the chilli/chile, ginger and garlic mixture to the pan. Cook for a further 5 minutes, stirring regularly. Remove from the heat, add the garam masala and the chopped coriander/cilantro and set to one side to cool.

To each spring roll wrapper, apply a dab of water along two conjoining sides. Add some filling and fold the wrapper in half, so that the wet sides sticks to the dry ones to form triangles. Press the together to firmly seal. Repeat for the rest of the wrappers and filling. Put the samosas on a baking sheet and refrigerate until needed.

Preheat the oil in a deep fat fryer or deep-sided saucepan to 180°C (350°F). Once it is ready, carefully lower the samosas in a few at a time and cook for about 5 minutes until golden brown. Drain on paper towels before serving.

CAULI EMPANADAS

These empanadas are perfect for feeding a crowd. Stuffed with olives, feta and vegetables with turmeric and paprika spiked pastry, they have a slightly Mediterranean feel and would be perfect for a summer party.

MAKES 12

PASTRY
375 g/generous 2¾ cups plain/
    all-purpose flour, plus extra for
    dusting
1 tablespoon smoked paprika
1 teaspoon ground turmeric
¼ teaspoon salt
225 g/1 cup butter, chilled and cubed
2 eggs, beaten

FILLING
2 tablespoons olive oil
1 onion, chopped
1 red (bell) pepper deseeded and,
    chopped
1 garlic clove, finely chopped
2 tablespoons freshly chopped
    oregano leaves
250 g/9 oz. cauliflower, trimmed
    and chopped
60 g/⅓ cup chopped pitted green
    olives
100 g/3½ oz. feta cheese, crumbled
2 egg yolks
20 g/generous 2 tablespoons
    sunflower seeds
salt and freshly ground black
    pepper

2 baking sheets, lined

Mix together the flour, paprika, turmeric and salt in a large bowl. Rub in the butter with your fingertips until crumbly. Stir in the eggs, then slowly add 3 tablespoons of cold water to bring the dough together. Turn onto a lightly floured surface and knead until smooth. Wrap the dough in clingfilm/plastic wrap and refrigerate for at least 1 hour.

Meanwhile, heat the olive oil in a frying pan/skillet over a medium-high heat. Add the onion, (bell) pepper, some salt and pepper and cook, stirring, for 5 minutes. Add the garlic and oregano and cook for 1 minute more. Cool.

Preheat the oven to 180°C (350°F) Gas 4. Divide the pastry dough into 12 portions and roll each one out into a thin round. Stir the cauliflower, olives and feta into the onion mixture. Place about 2½ tablespoons of vegetable filling in the centre of each pastry circle. Wet the edges of the pastry, then fold in half and pinch the sides together to seal. Use a fork to crimp the edges. Make a few small slits on top of each empanada and transfer to the prepared baking sheets. Whisk the egg yolks with 2 tablespoons of water. Brush the tops of the empanadas with the egg wash and top with sunflower seeds. Bake in the preheated oven for 25–30 minutes until golden brown.

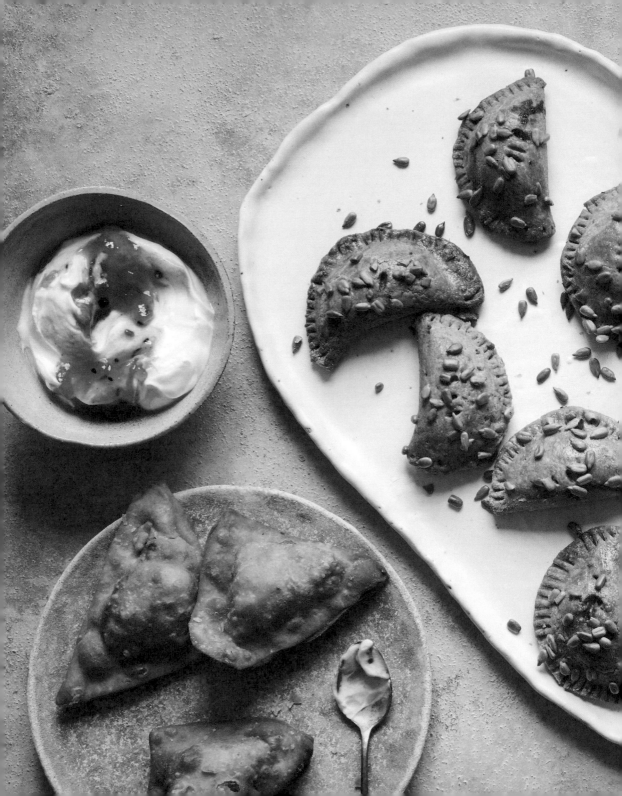

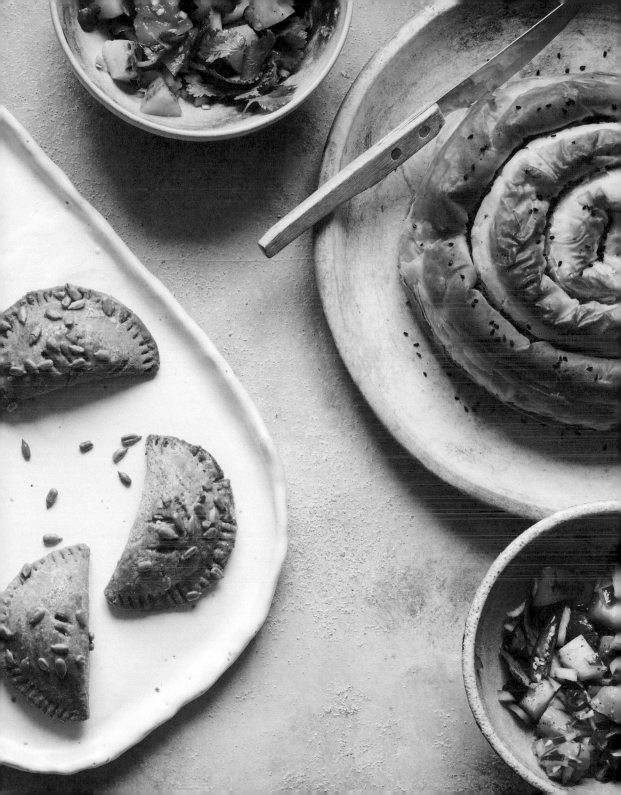

CAULI & FETA SWIRL

SERVES 4–6

1 cauliflower, trimmed
1 tablespoon extra-virgin olive oil
2 garlic cloves, finely chopped
3 spring onions/scallions, finely chopped
200 g/7 oz. feta, crumbled
3 eggs, lightly beaten
handful of mint, leaves picked
75 g/⅓ cup butter, melted
8 sheets filo/Phyllo pastry
1 tablespoon nigella seeds
salt and freshly ground black pepper

23-cm/9-inch cake pan

Pulse the cauliflower in a food processor to roughly chop. Heat the oil in a pan/skillet over a medium-high heat. Fry the cauliflower for 5 minutes until golden. Add the garlic and spring onions/scallions. Transfer to a bowl and let cool. Add the feta, eggs and mint and season.

Preheat the oven to 200°C (400°F) Gas 6.

Brush the pan with melted butter. Brush one pastry sheet with butter, then top with another sheet. Brush with more butter. Place a quarter of the cauli mix along the long side closest to you. Fold in the sides and roll up. Shape into a coil, seam-side down in the centre of the pan. Repeat to make three more rolls and wrap around to fill the pan. Brush with melted butter. Bake on lowest shelf for 30 minutes. Transfer to the middle shelf and bake for 15–20 minutes more until golden. Top with nigella seeds.

QUINOA & CAULI MINI CAKES

MAKES 12

150 g/5½ oz. quinoa
100 g/3½ oz. cauliflower, blitzed
1 large beetroot/beet, peeled and grated
60 g/2¼ oz. thinly sliced spring onion/scallion
1 small red onion, finely diced
2 eggs, lightly beaten
2 green chillies/chiles, deseeded and finely diced
120 g/generous ½ cup cottage cheese
50 g/1¾ oz. crumbled feta
60 g/¾ cup dried breadcrumbs
1 teaspoon smoked paprika
60 ml/¼ cup olive oil
grated zest and freshly squeezed juice of 1 lemon
yogurt, with extra smoked paprika stirred in and micro cress, to garnish

muffin pan, greased or lined with paper cases

Preheat the oven to 180°C (350°F) Gas 4.

Bring a pan of water to the boil, add the quinoa and simmer for 11 minutes, until al dente. Drain, then refresh in cold water and squeeze out the liquid.

Put the rest of the ingredients into a bowl along with the quinoa and mix well to combine. Divide the mixture between the greased or lined holes of the muffin pan and then bake in the preheated oven for 30 minutes. Serve with paprika yogurt and garnished with micro cress.

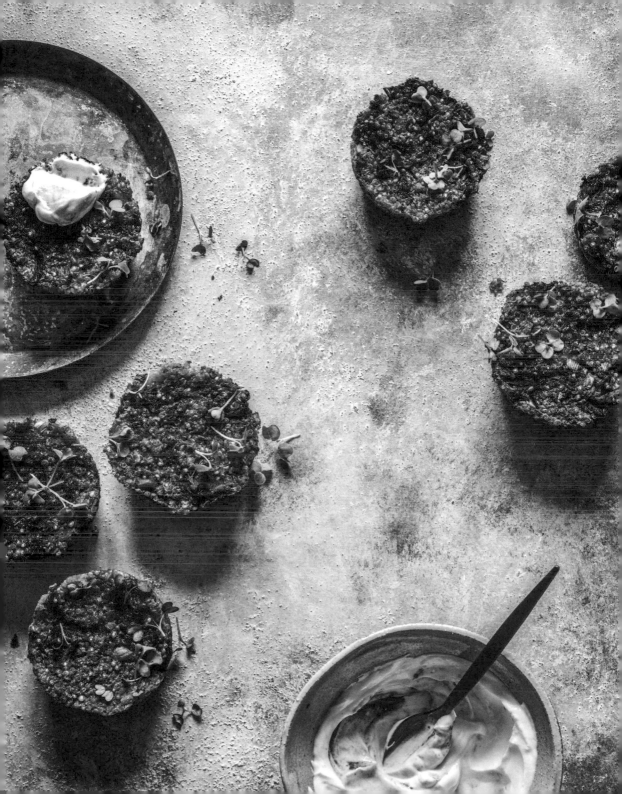

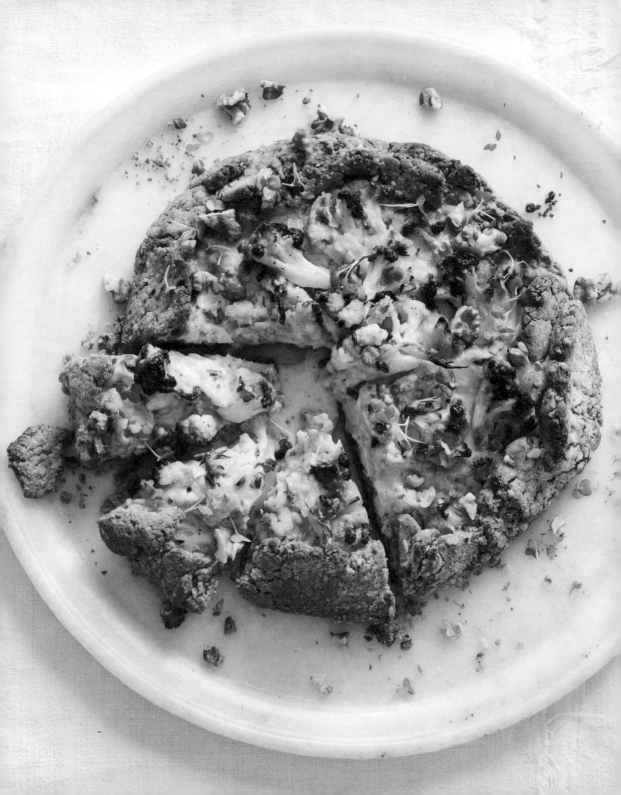

FREEFORM CAULIFLOWER PIE WITH WALNUT & OAT PASTRY

This rustic freeform pie is a wonderfully comforting main dish.
Serve with a crisp side salad and an equally crisp glass of Chardonnay.

SERVES 4

PASTRY
200 g/1¹/₂ cups plain/all-purpose
    flour, plus extra for dusting
50 g/¹/₃ cup walnuts
20 g/scant ¹/₄ cup rolled/
    old-fashioned oats
60 g/¹/₄ cup butter
25 g/1 oz. grated Parmesan or other
    vegetarian hard cheese
1 UK large/US extra-large egg,
    beaten

CAULIFLOWER FILLING
1 tablespoon olive oil
4 shallots, thinly sliced
2 garlic cloves, crushed
1 whole cauliflower, trimmed and
    roughly chopped
4 sprigs fresh thyme, leaves picked
150 g/5¹/₂ oz. vegetarian taleggio,
    rind removed
100 ml/scant ¹/₂ cup double/heavy
    cream
1 teaspoon Dijon mustard
¹/₂ bunch chives, finely chopped
salt and freshly ground black
    pepper

TO GARNISH
1 tablespoon toasted walnuts,
    roughly chopped
cress

For the pastry, combine the flour, walnuts and oats in a food processor and process to very fine crumbs. Add the butter and cheese and process again until the mixture resembles breadcrumbs. Add the beaten egg and 1–2 teaspoon(s) of cold water. Pulse until the mixture comes together into a dough, adding a little more water if needed. Wrap in cling film/plastic wrap and refrigerate for 30 minutes.

For the filling, heat the oil in a frying pan/skillet over a medium-high heat. Add the shallots and fry, stirring, for 10 minutes or until golden. Add the garlic and cook, stirring, for 1 minute. Add the chopped cauliflower and cook, stirring, for 10 minutes or until just tender. Transfer to a bowl and leave to cool slightly. Add the thyme, taleggio, cream, Dijon mustard and chives. Season to taste and set aside.

Preheat the oven to 200°C (400°F) Gas 6, with a baking sheet inside.

Dust a large sheet of baking parchment with a little flour, then roll out the pastry on top of this into a rough circle, about 30 cm/12 inches wide. Arrange the cauliflower filling in the centre of the pastry, leaving a clear border of roughly 5 cm/2 inches all the way around. Season with salt and pepper, then fold up the pastry edges to partly enclose the filling. Transfer the tart to the preheated baking sheet, using the paper. Bake in the preheated oven for 30 minutes until the pastry is golden. Garnish with extra walnuts and sprinkle with cress. Eat just warm or at room temperature.

CAULIFLOWER, VEGETABLE & BEAN RAGÙ ⓥ

This will become your staple tomato ragù. Keep a batch in the freezer ready to add to your chilli, swirl through pasta, or serve instead of home made baked beans for brunch.

MAKES 2.5 KG/5¹/₂ LB (PERFECT TO FREEZE)

2 onions, diced
2 carrots, diced
2 sticks celery, diced
2 heads of cauliflower, cut into florets
1 large aubergine/eggplant, diced
2 tablespoons olive oil
a few sprigs each fresh thyme, rosemary and sage
2 fresh bay leaves
100 ml/¹/₃ cup vegan red wine
2 x 400-g/14-oz. cans good-quality plum tomatoes
400-g/14-oz. can haricot/navy beans, drained and rinsed
salt and freshly ground black pepper

For the ragù, place the onions, carrots, celery, cauliflower and aubergine/eggplant in a large, flameproof casserole dish with the olive oil. Cook over a medium heat for 20 minutes, or until softened, stirring often, as the veg sticks easily.

Tie the herb sprigs and bay leaves together with string/twine to make a bouquet garni and add to the pan. After a few minutes, pour in the wine and leave to bubble and cook away for about. 3–5 minutes.

Tip in the tomatoes, breaking them up with the back of a wooden spoon, then pour in two cans of water. Cook for 30 minutes, then add the beans. Cook for 30 minutes more, or until thickened and reduced, stirring and mashing occasionally with a potato masher, and adding splashes of water to loosen, if needed.

Season to taste with salt and pepper before serving.

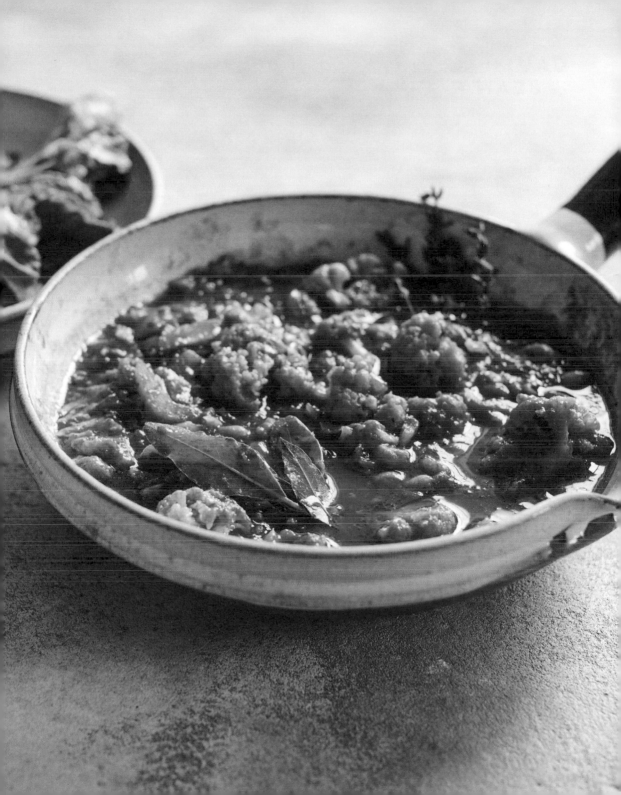

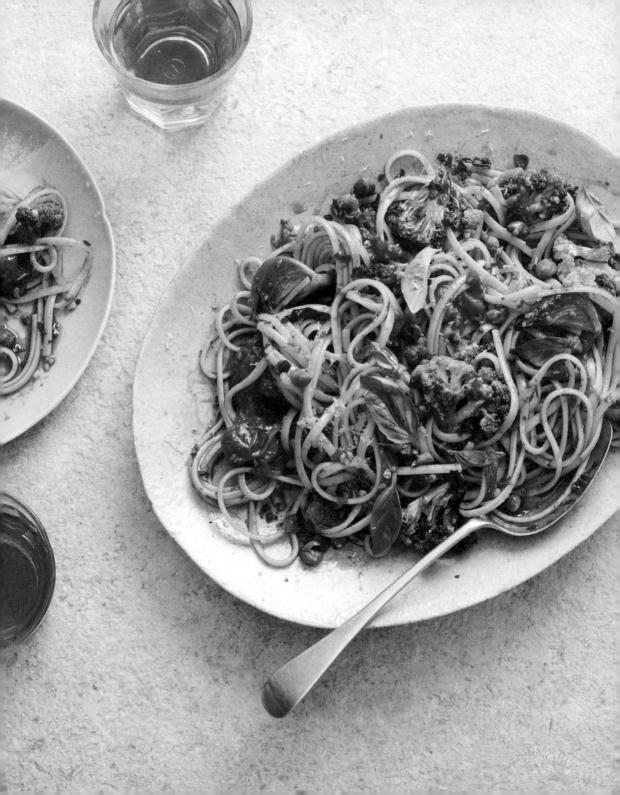

LINGUINE WITH SMASHED CAULI, TOMATO, HARISSA & CAPERS Ⓥ

The simplicity of this recipe is second to none, and the oven does most of the work for you. But finishing the dish with tart and salty capers and feta, fresh basil and zingy lemon zest leads to a taste sensation.

SERVES 2

1 whole cauliflower, trimmed
   and cut into florets
3 large tomatoes
6 garlic cloves, unpeeled
4 tablespoons olive oil
200 g/7 oz. dried linguine pasta
3 tablespoons harissa paste
2 tablespoons capers, drained
handful of fresh basil leaves
grated zest of 1 lemon (optional)
salt and freshly ground black
   pepper

*large roasting pan, lined with
   baking parchment*

Preheat the oven to 160°C (325°F) Gas 3.

Place the cauliflower, tomatoes and garlic cloves in the prepared roasting pan. Drizzle with 3 tablespoons of the olive oil, season with salt and pepper and lightly toss to combine. Roast in the preheated oven for about 40 minutes until the vegetables have coloured and are quite soft.

Crush/smash the roasted cauliflower and tomatoes with a fork in a bowl. Press the garlic cloves out of their skins and mash through with a fork, then mix into the cauli and tomatoes. Keep warm in a low oven. Alternatively, if you want a smooth sauce with your pasta, you could blitz the roasted veg and garlic in a food processor with the cooking juices to create a vegetable sauce, and keep warm over the lowest heat on the hob/stovetop.

Bring a large saucepan of salted water to the boil and cook the linguine according to the packet instructions. Drain and then return to the saucepan. Stir the remaining 1 tablespoon olive oil, the harissa paste and roasted cauli, tomatoes and garlic mixture into the hot pasta.

Divide into serving bowls or serve on a large platter. Finish by topping with the capers, basil leaves and lemon zest, if you like.

BEER-BATTERED CAULIFLOWER & SHOESTRING COURGETTE FRIES

Carry the flavour through and serve with an ice-cold beer – a perfect
alternative to fish and chips on a Friday.

SERVES 4

750 ml–1 litre/3–4 cups
    vegetable oil
225 g/1³⁄₄ cups self-raising/
    rising flour
360 ml/1¹⁄₂ cups lager
1 cauliflower, cut into florets
plain/all-purpose flour, seasoned,
    for dusting
salt and freshly ground black
    pepper
lemon wedges, to serve

SHOESTRING COURGETTE/ ZUCCHINI FRIES

3 large courgettes/zucchini
about 400 ml/1³⁄₄ cups cold milk
about 400 g/3 cups plain/
    all-purpose flour, seasoned

Preheat the oil in a deep fat fryer or deep-sided saucepan
to 180°C (350°F). When a cube of bread dropped in sizzles,
browns and rises to the surface, then it should be ready.

For the beer batter, place the self-raising/rising flour
in a bowl and whisk in the lager until a smooth batter forms.

Dust the cauliflower with seasoned flour, dusting off any
excess, then dip in the batter, shaking off any excess.
Deep-fry in batches, turning occasionally with a slotted
spoon, until crisp and cooked through, about 3–4 minutes
(be careful as hot oil may spit). Drain on paper towels and
keep warm until ready to serve.

For the shoestring courgette/zucchini fries, finely julienne
the courgettes/zucchini to make strings.

Carefully dredge the courgette/zucchini strings in the
milk, then drain and shake around in the seasoned flour
to lightly coat.

Lower the courgette/zucchini fries into the hot oil in
batches and cook for 3 minutes or until light golden brown.
Remove using a slotted spoon and leave to drain on paper
towels. Keep warm until ready to serve.

Serve the beer-battered cauliflower and courgette/zucchini
fries with wedges of lemon and plenty of salt and pepper.

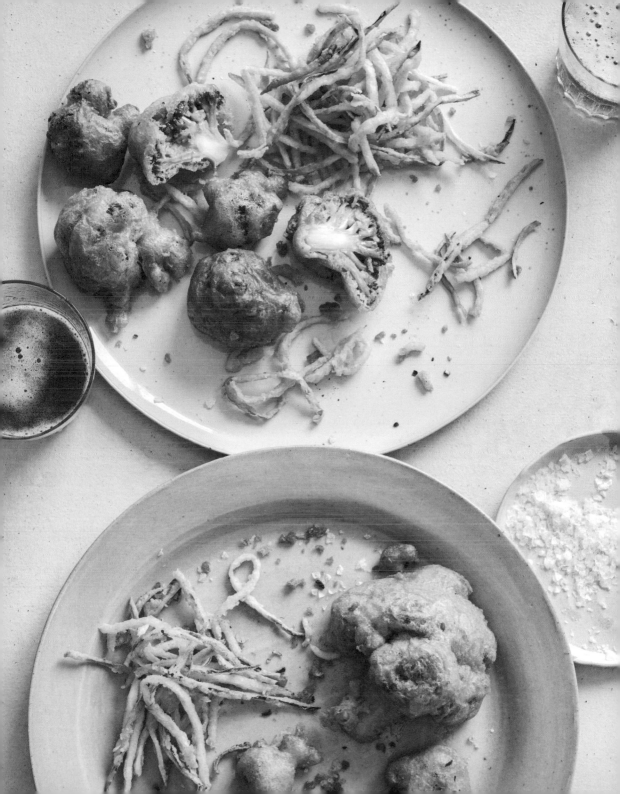

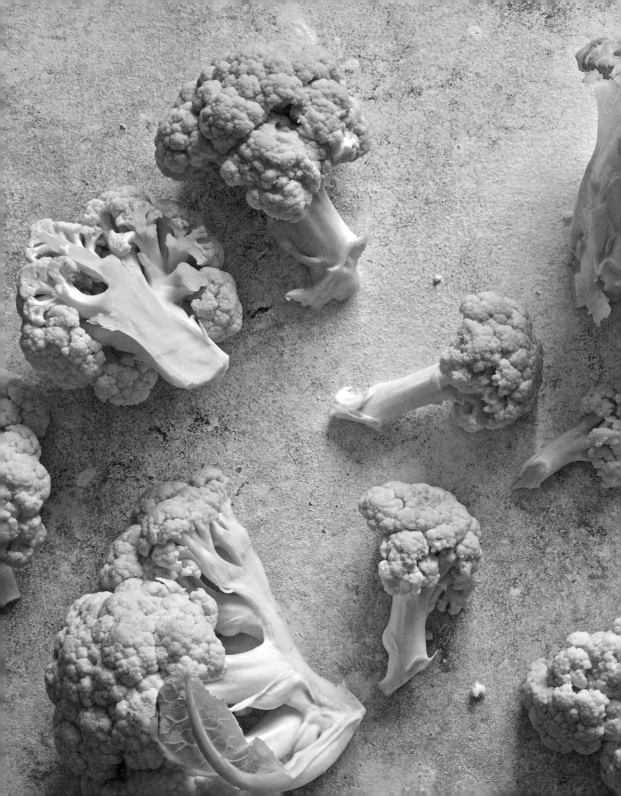

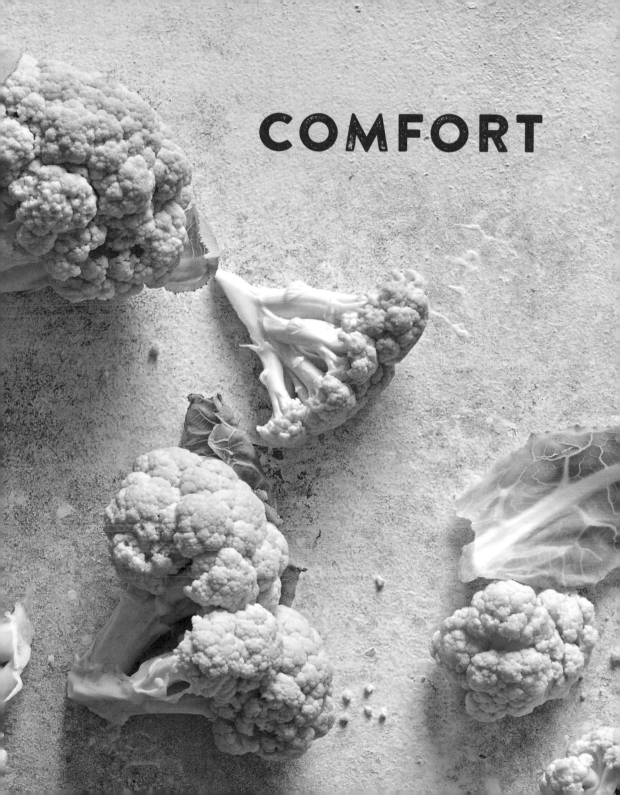

COMFORT

CAULI CORNBREAD WITH GREEN CHILLI & GARLIC BUTTER

I love to eat this cornbread warm, slathered in the green chilli/chile and garlic butter, or toasted under the grill/broiler with soup, or topped with a fried egg. There are so many ways to devour this!

SERVES 4–6

300 g/10½ oz. cauliflower, cut into florets
4 tablespoons olive oil
2 leeks, thinly sliced
260 g/1¾ cups cornmeal/polenta
280 g/generous 2 cups self-raising/ self-rising flour
2 teaspoons baking powder
1 teaspoon bicarbonate of soda/ baking soda
1 teaspoon salt
150 g/5½ oz. goat's cheese
50 g/scant ⅔ cups coarsely grated vegetarian hard cheese
80 g/3 oz. garlic chives or normal chives, chopped
500 g/2⅓ cups Greek yogurt
3 eggs

GREEN CHILLI/CHILE & GARLIC BUTTER

100 g/7 tablespoons salted butter
1 green chilli/chile, chopped
20 g/¾ oz. wild garlic/ramps or 3 garlic cloves, crushed

1 x round 23-cm/9-inch cake pan, greased and lined

Steam the cauliflower for 10 minutes, then remove from the heat and set aside to cool. It can be pre-cooked and kept cold in the fridge, if you wish.

Heat 2 tablespoons of the oil in a pan over a medium heat. Sauté the leeks for 5 minutes, stirring frequently. Set aside to cool.

Preheat the oven to 190°C (375°F) Gas 5.

Combine the cornmeal/polenta, flour, baking powder, bicarbonate of soda/baking soda, salt, both cheeses, chives, cauliflower and cooled leeks in a large mixing bowl. Toss gently to mix well.

In another bowl, whisk together the yogurt, eggs and remaining 2 tablespoons of oil. Pour this over the dry ingredients and mix well to combine. Spoon the mixture into the prepared baking pan and bake in the preheated oven for 30–40 minutes, or until golden and cooked through.

Remove from the baking pan when cool enough to handle. The cornbread can be eaten at room temperature, but is best eaten when warm.

To make the green chilli/chile and garlic butter, process all the ingredients together in a food processor until smooth. Chill in the fridge for 10 minutes to firm up and then serve with the cornbread.

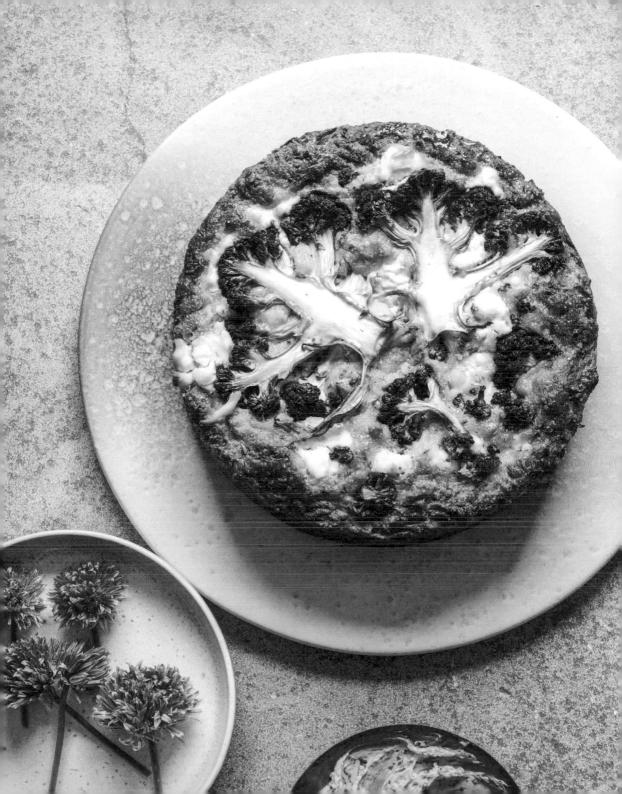

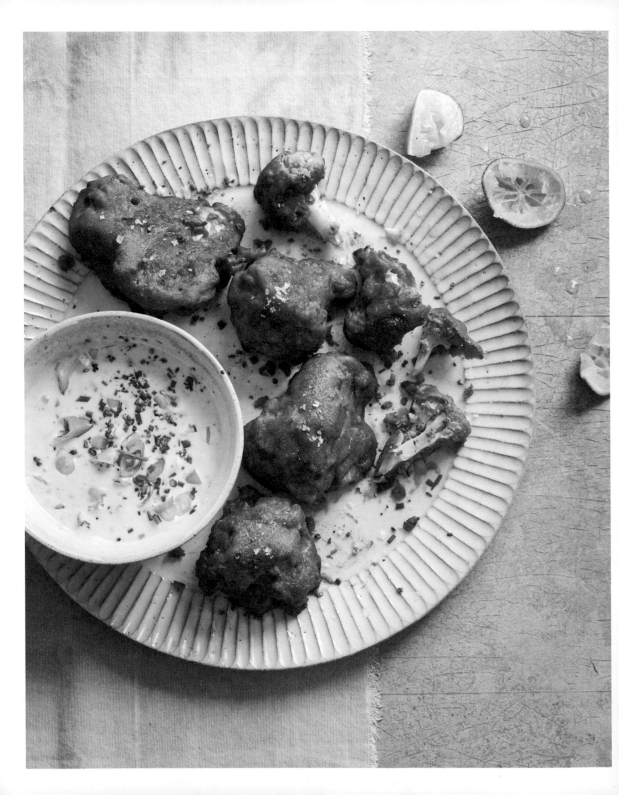

CAULIFLOWER BUFFALO WINGS Ⓥ

Inspired by the traditionally deep-fried American buffalo wings, these cauliflower 'wings' are coated in Frank's red hot sauce and then baked to create a moreish, sweet and spicy vegan version of the classic.

SERVES 4 AS AN APPETIZER

150–180 ml/^{2}/$_3$–^{3}/$_4$ cup almond
  or soy milk
150 g/generous 1 cup plain/
  all-purpose flour
2 teaspoons garlic powder
1 teaspoon ground cumin
1 teaspoon paprika
1 cauliflower, cut into 'wing'-size
  florets
2 tablespoons vegan butter
100 ml/^{1}/$_3$ cup Frank's red hot sauce
  (or other chilli/hot sauce)
freshly squeezed juice of 1 lime
salt and freshly ground black
  pepper

TO SERVE
lime wedges
vegan ranch-style dressing or vegan
  yogurt
snipped chives and sliced spring
  onions/scallions (optional)

baking sheet, lined

Preheat the oven to 200°C (400°F) Gas 6.

Mix the milk, flour and spices in a medium mixing bowl. Mix until the batter is thick and is able to coat the cauliflower without dripping.

Dip the cauliflower florets in the batter one by one. Shake off any excess batter before placing the cauliflower on the lined baking sheet in a single layer.

Bake in the preheated oven for 20 minutes until golden brown, flipping the florets over halfway through to get all sides golden brown and crispy.

While the cauliflower is baking, get your buffalo wing sauce ready. In a small saucepan over a low heat, melt all of the butter and mix in the hot sauce. Remove from the heat just as it starts to melt. Stir together and set aside.

Once the cauliflower has finished its first bake in the batter, remove it from the oven and put all the baked florets into a mixing bowl with the wing sauce and toss to coat evenly. Return the cauliflower to the baking sheet and bake in the oven for another 10–15 minutes or until it has reached the desired crispness.

Serve with extra seasoning, lime wedges for squeezing over and cooling vegan ranch-style dressing or vegan yogurt for dipping. Garnish the dip with snipped chives and spring/onions scallions, if you like.

CAULIFLOWER SKEWERS WITH PIRI PIRI SAUCE

This fiery piri-piri sauce is the perfect condiment for these skewers. The combination of the saltness of the halloumi, freshness of the mint and the earthy cauliflower will become one of your favourites.

SERVES 4

1 cauliflower, cut into florets
200 g/7 oz. halloumi, cut into
    5-cm/2-inch cubes
1 bunch asparagus, cut into thirds
1 bunch spring onions/scallions, cut
    into thirds
½ bunch mint, leaves picked
2 tablespoons olive oil
freshly squeezed juice of 1 lemon
salt and freshly ground black pepper

PIRI PIRI SAUCE

2 red onions, roughly chopped
6 garlic cloves, chopped
2 red chillies/chiles, chopped
2 red (bell) peppers, roughly chopped
3 ripe tomatoes, roughly chopped
4 tablespoons olive oil
grated zest and freshly squeezed
    juice of 3 lemons
100 ml/⅓ cup red wine vinegar
2 tablespoons soft brown sugar
1 tablespoon salt
1 teaspoon ground black pepper
1 tablespoon dried oregano
1 tablespoon smoked paprika
2 bay leaves

8 wooden skewers, soaked in water
    for 30 minutes

To make the piri piri sauce (this will make extra but if you are going to make the effort you may as well make more), combine all the ingredients except the bay leaves in the bowl of a food processor, and mix until finely chopped and the mixture has a sauce-like consistency.

Transfer to a saucepan over a medium heat and add the bay leaves. Simmer for 30–40 minutes, stirring every few minutes to prevent the sauce from burning. After 20 minutes, check the seasoning and adjust. The sauce should be well balanced with a good kick of spice and sourness from the lemon and vinegar. Discard the bay leaves. Pour into sterilized jars/bottles, seal and keep in the fridge for up to 2 weeks.

For the skewers, preheat the grill/broiler to high or alternatively heat a griddle/grill pan to high.

Thread and divide the cauliflower, halloumi cubes, asparagus, spring onions/scallions and mint leaves between the soaked wooden skewers. Brush with the olive oil and season with salt and pepper and the lemon juice.

Cook under the grill/broiler for 10–12 minutes, or until the cheese is golden and the vegetables are soft, turning halfway through. If cooking in a griddle/grill pan, cook on each side for 4–5 minutes. Serve the skewers with the piri piri sauce for dipping.

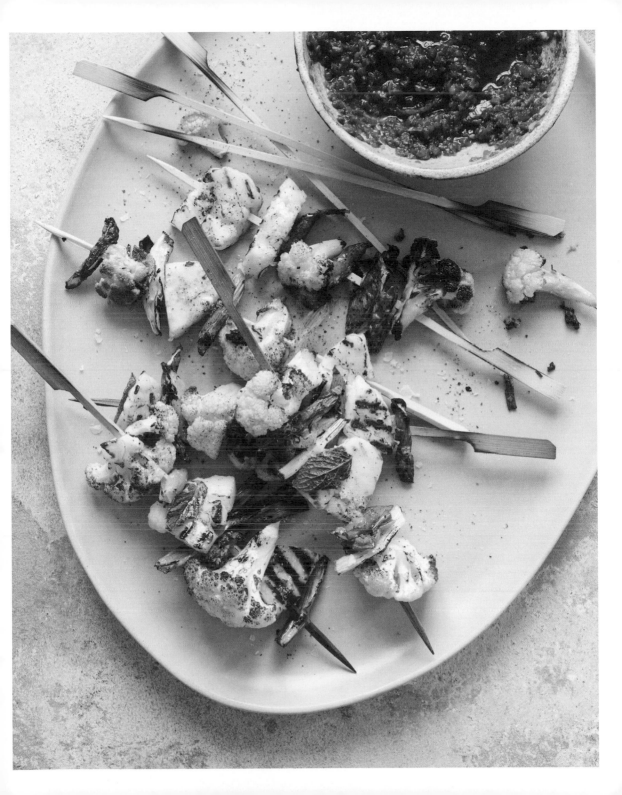

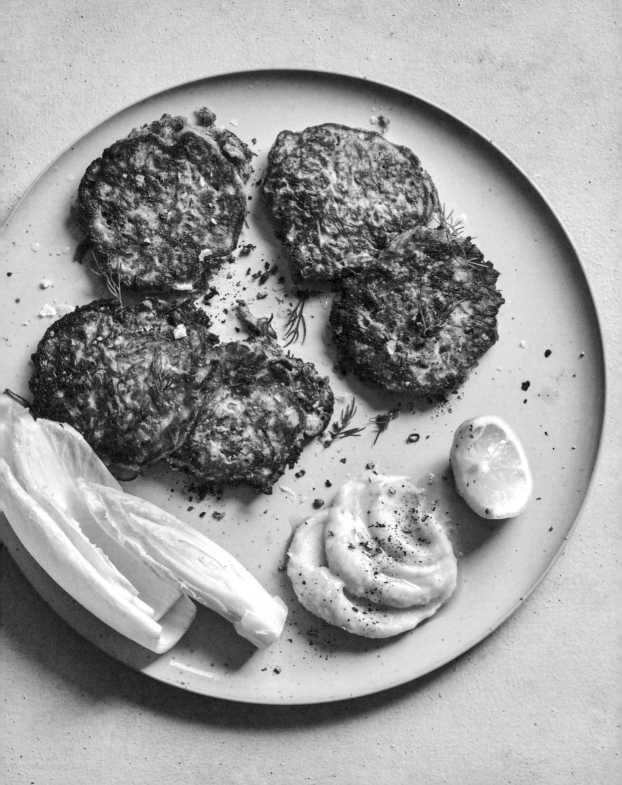

FLUFFY CAULIFLOWER & DILL FRITTERS WITH SKORDALIA

This recipe is great for lunch, or for little ones as a finger food snack.
Served with skordalia – a tangy garlic sauce – they are delicious!

MAKES 12

FRITTERS
1 large red onion, coarsely diced
2 tablespoons olive oil, plus
 100–150 ml/$^1/_3$–$^2/_3$ cup olive oil,
 for deep-frying
400 g/14 oz. cauliflower, grated
 or blitzed coarsely in a food
 processor
3 eggs
125 g/1 cup plain/all-purpose flour
1 tablespoon freshly chopped mint
 leaves
2 tablespoons freshly chopped dill,
 plus extra spigs to garnish
salt and freshly ground black
 pepper
lemon wedges, to serve
salad garnish such as chicory/
 endive leaves

LEMON SKORDALIA
1 medium potato (about 200 g/
 7 oz.), quartered
6 garlic cloves (left in their skins
 and roasted in foil)
grated zest and freshly squeezed
 juice of 2 lemons
80 ml/$^1/_3$ cup olive oil, plus extra
 for drizzling

For the skordalia, boil, steam or microwave the potato until tender, then drain. Push it through a food mill or fine sieve/strainer into a large bowl; let cool for 10 minutes. Add the garlic flesh, lemon juice and 2 tablespoons of cold water, and stir until well combined. Place the potato mixture in a blender, then, with the motor running, gradually add the oil in a thin, steady stream, blending only until the skordalia thickens (do not overmix). Add the lemon zest, spoon into a bowl and drizzle with extra oil.

For the fritters, in a large frying pan/skillet, fry the onion in the olive oil over a medium heat for 5 minutes until it is soft and lightly coloured. Add the cauliflower and sauté for 2 minutes, stirring. Tip into a sieve/strainer to drain off any excess liquid and allow to cool slightly.

In a bowl, whisk the eggs with the flour until well blended. Mix in the herbs and some black pepper, together with the cooked onion and cauliflower. If the batter is too runny, add a little more flour.

Put a large, non-stick frying pan/skillet over a medium heat and add enough olive oil to deep-fry the fritters. Heat until a cube of bread dropped in sizzles and rises to the top. Spoon in dollops of the batter, in batches. Turn and cook until both sides are lightly browned. Drain on paper towels.

Season and serve with the skordalia, lemon wedges, extra dill sprigs and a salad garnish such as chicory/endive leaves.

CREAMY CAULI MASH

This creamy cauli tastes like mashed potatoes but is much lower in carbohydrates – the perfect side dish.

SERVES 4

1 cauliflower, cut into medium florets
2–3 tablespoons double/heavy cream
15 g/1 tablespoon butter, plus extra to serve
1 tablespoon grated Parmesan or other vegetarian hard cheese, plus extra to serve
1/4 teaspoon freshly grated nutmeg
salt and freshly ground black pepper

Place the cauliflower in a steamer basket set over a large pan of 2.5 cm/1 inch of simmering water. Cover and steam for 6–8 minutes, until fork tender.

Drain the steamed cauliflower and transfer to the bowl of a large food processor while still warm. Add the remaining ingredients and blitz until it reaches the desired consistency (the smoother it is, the better it will hold together).

Test the seasoning and serve with extra butter and cheese for extra indulgence.

CREAMY VEGAN CAULI MASH Ⓥ

Everyone will love this dreamy, herby vegan mash, it is not just for vegans.

SERVES 4

1 cauliflower, cut into medium florets
100 ml/1/3 cup vegan cream (such as oat cream)
3 roasted garlic cloves, peeled
1 teaspoon fresh thyme leaves
1 teaspoon fresh snipped chives
salt and freshly ground black pepper

Place the cauliflower in a steamer basket set over a large pan of 2.5 cm/1 inch of simmering water. Cover and steam for 6–8 minutes, until fork tender.

Drain the steamed cauliflower and transfer to the bowl of a large food processor while still warm. Add the remaining ingredients and process to your desired consistency.

CELERIAC & CAULI MASH WITH CAULI CROUTONS

A luxurious, impressive mash with the delicate flavour of celeriac.

SERVES 4

1 cauliflower, chopped (reserving 3 florets)
1 celeriac, peeled and roughly chopped
2–3 roasted garlic cloves, peeled
50 g/3½ tablespoons butter
salt and freshly ground black pepper

CAULI CROUTONS

3 reserved cauliflower florets
½ teaspoon celery salt
¼ teaspoon ground black pepper
1 tablespoon olive oil
1 celery stick, shaved lengthways, to serve
3 sprigs chervil, leaves picked, to serve
freshly squeezed juice of ½ lemon, to serve

Place the cauliflower and celeriac in a steamer basket set over a large pan of 2.5 cm/1 inch of simmering water. Cover and steam for 6–8 minutes, until tender. Drain and transfer to a food processor. Add the garlic, butter and some seasoning. Blend until smooth.

Preheat the oven to 190°C (375°F) Gas 5.

Place the reserved cauli on a lined baking sheet. Season with the celery salt and pepper and top with the olive oil. Bake in the oven for 20–30 minutes until crisp. Top the mash with the cauli croutons, celery, chervil and lemon juice.

VELVET CAULI WHIPPED MASH

The addition of potato to the cauli makes for a super smooth, light velvety mash.

SERVES 4

1 cauliflower, trimmed and chopped
1 large potato, peeled and chopped
1 garlic clove, peeled
500 ml/2 cups vegetable stock
1 bay leaf
50 g/3½ tablespoons butter
2 tablespoons double/heavy cream
salt and freshly ground black pepper

PARSLEY & GARLIC OIL

30 g/1 oz. flat leaf parsley
60 ml/¼ cup extra virgin olive oil
zest of 1 lemon and ½ tablespoon lemon juice
3 large cloves garlic

Combine all the parsley and garlic oil ingredients in a food processor and pulse to make a smooth sauce.

Place the cauliflower, potato and garlic with the vegetable stock and bay leaf in a large pot. Cover with a lid and cook for 10–12 minutes until the vegetables are tender. Discard the bay leaf and drain off the stock and discard.

Mash the cauliflower and potato until smooth, then add the butter and cream and season. Serve swirled with the parsley and garlic oil. Leftovers will keep in the fridge for up to a week.

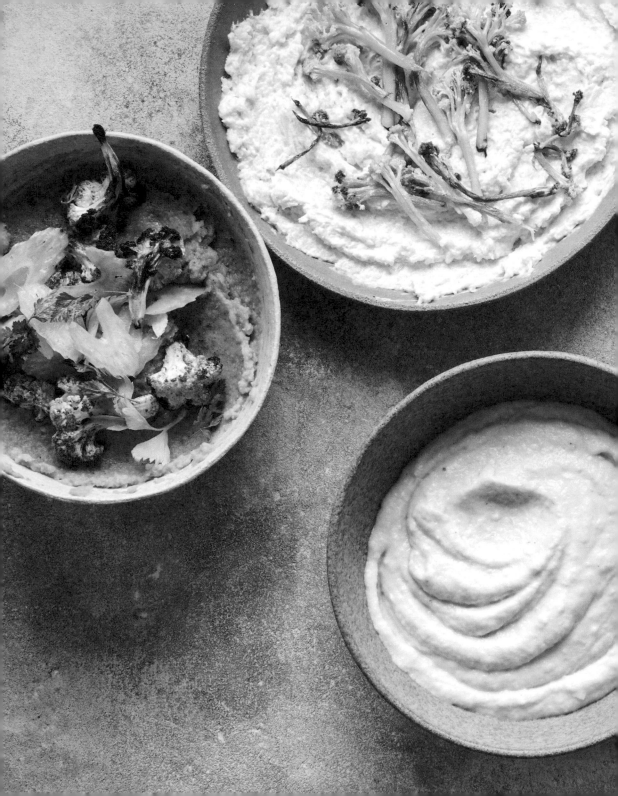

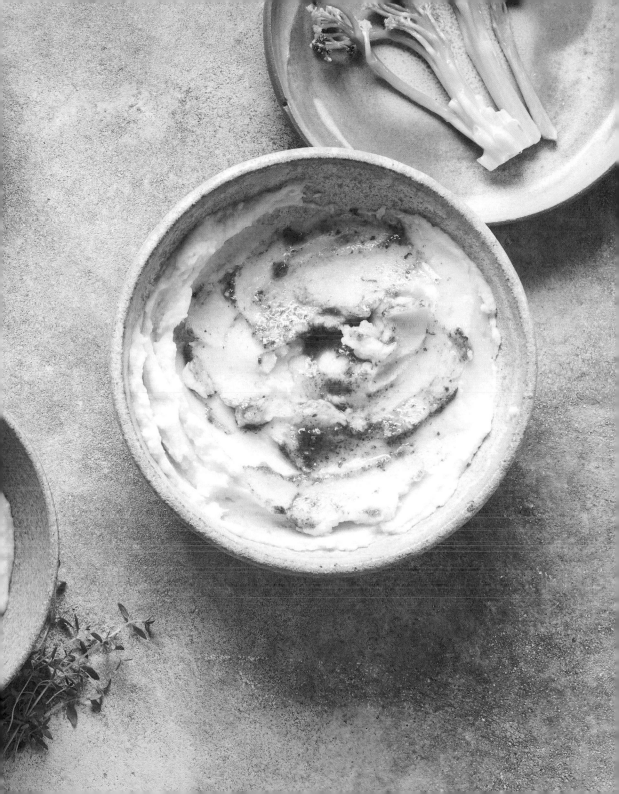

SPICED CAULIFLOWER TACOS

Give these spicy vegetarian tacos a try. They are super easy to make and great for a fun, relaxed meal.

SERVES 2–3

1 cauliflower
1 teaspoon chilli/chili powder
1 teaspoon smoked paprika
1 teaspoon ground cumin
1 teaspoon onion powder
1 teaspoon garlic powder
1/4 teaspoon cayenne pepper
   (optional)
large pinch of salt
2 tablespoons olive oil

TO SERVE
tortillas, warmed
sour cream with chipotle in adobo
coriander/cilantro leaves
sliced red cabbage
sliced red onions
sliced avocado
lime wedges

baking sheet, lined

Preheat the oven to 200°C (400°F) Gas 6.

While the oven is heating, chop the cauliflower into bite-sized florets and stir together the spices with the salt in a small bowl.

Put the cauliflower in a large mixing bowl and lightly coat it with the olive oil.

Sprinkle the spice mix over the top of the cauliflower and gently toss again to coat each floret evenly with the spices.

Spread the spiced cauliflower onto the lined baking sheet and bake in the preheated oven for about 25 minutes.

While the cauliflower is cooking, prepare all of your desired taco accompaniments.

Once the cauliflower is ready, simply fill your warmed tortillas, add the accompaniments of your choice and finish with a squeeze of fresh lime juice.

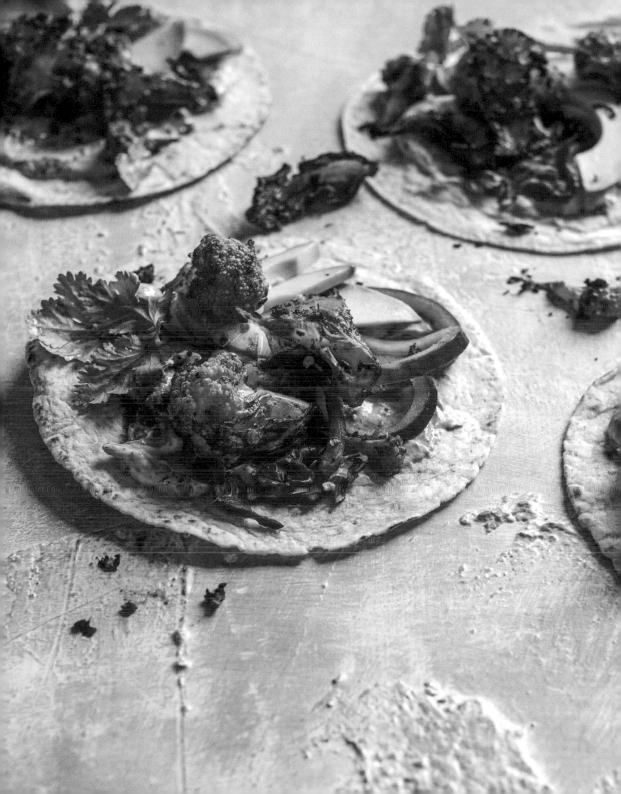

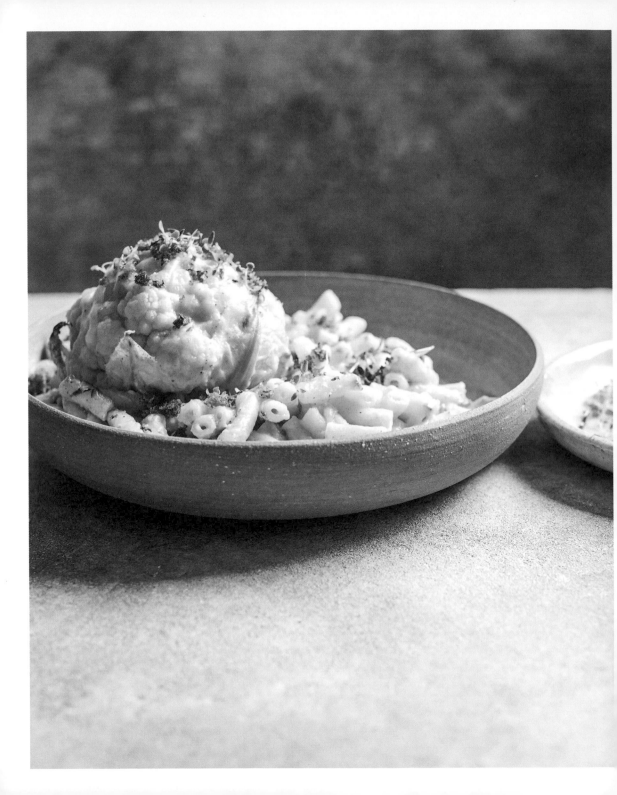

MINI ROASTED CAULIFLOWER CHEESE ON A MACARONI BASE WITH A ZESTY THYME CRUMB

Mac 'n' cheese is always a winner. With the addition of cauliflower and a crumb, it is transformed into a more nutritious and sophisticated meal.

SERVES 4

250 g/9 oz. mini macaroni

4 mini cauliflowers or 1 whole cauliflower, cut into 4 wedges

25 g/2 tablespoons butter

2 tablespoons plain/all-purpose flour

2 teaspoons wholegrain mustard

450 ml/scant 2 cups full-fat/whole milk

100 g/generous 1 cup grated Cheddar cheese

1 tablespoon snipped chives

40 g/1/3 cup semi-dried tomatoes, chopped (optional)

salt and freshly ground black pepper

ZESTY THYME CRUMB

15 g/1 tablespoon butter

40 g/2/3 cup fresh breadcrumbs (preferably sourdough)

4 sprigs lemon thyme, leaves picked

pinch of dried chilli flakes/hot red pepper flakes

grated zest of 1/2 lemon

Cook the macaroni according to the packet instructions, adding the cauliflowers for the final 4 minutes.

Meanwhile, make the zesty thyme crumb. In a frying pan/ skillet, gently heat the butter, then add the breadcrumbs and cook until they are a toasty colour, about 5 minutes. Remove from the heat and stir in the lemon thyme, chilli flakes/hot red pepper flakes and lemon zest. Set aside.

Melt the butter in a pan, then stir in the flour and mustard and cook for 2 minutes. Gradually add the milk, stirring all the time to get a smooth sauce. Add three-quarters of the cheese and some seasoning.

Drain the macaroni and cauliflower and stir into the cheese sauce, adding the snipped chives and semi-dried tomatoes (if using). Transfer to an ovenproof dish, then sprinkle over the remaining cheese and the zesty crumb. Flash under a preheated hot grill/broiler until golden and bubbling. Serve with a green salad, if you like.

CAULIFLOWER GNOCCHI WITH ASPARAGUS & PEAS

Cauliflower and ricotta make this gnocchi very light and soft. It is the perfect spring dish with vibrant green peas and asparagus.

SERVES 4

350 g/12 oz. cauliflower, cut into florets
100 g/1½ cups finely grated Parmesan or other vegetarian hard cheese
2 egg yolks
150 g/1 cup strong white flour
150 g/⅔ cup ricotta

ASPARAGUS & PEA SAUCE

140 ml/scant ⅔ cup double/heavy cream
1 garlic clove, crushed
1 bunch asparagus, halved lengthways
100 g/⅔ cup podded fresh peas
50 g/¾ cup finely grated Parmesan or other vegetarian hard cheese
pinch of freshly grated nutmeg
5 g/¼ cup (loosely packed) mint, leaves picked and chopped
5 g/¼ cup (loosely packed) parsley, leaves picked and chopped, plus extra to garnish
grated zest of 1 lemon, plus extra to garnish

baking sheet, lined

Place the cauliflower in a steamer and cook for about 15–20 minutes until tender, then blitz in a food processor. Add in the remaining ingredients, except the ricotta. Pulse until combined well. Then add the ricotta to the cauliflower mixture until all combined.

With wet fingers, form the mixture into gnocchi, using 1–2 teaspoons of batter for each one, depending on how big you want them. Continue to wet your fingers as you form each piece. Once formed, sit them on a wet fork and roll them over the fork. Place them on the lined baking sheet. Freeze for 1 hour or until ready to use. (Note: These are not as firm as regular potato gnocchi – you can add a few extra tablespoons of flour if you prefer a firmer texture, but I like them light and fluffy.)

Bring a pot of salted water to the boil. Place about 10–12 gnocchi at a time in the boiling water and cook for 2 minutes. Remove each batch using a slotted spoon and keep warm while you cook the remainder.

For the sauce, bring the cream and garlic to the boil in a small saucepan. Add the asparagus and fresh peas. Remove from the heat, then set the pan aside for 1–2 minutes for the veg to lightly cook. Add half the grated Parmesan or hard cheese, the nutmeg, mint, parsley and lemon zest. Mix the gnocchi into the sauce and serve, finished with the remaining cheese, extra mint leaves and grated lemon zest.

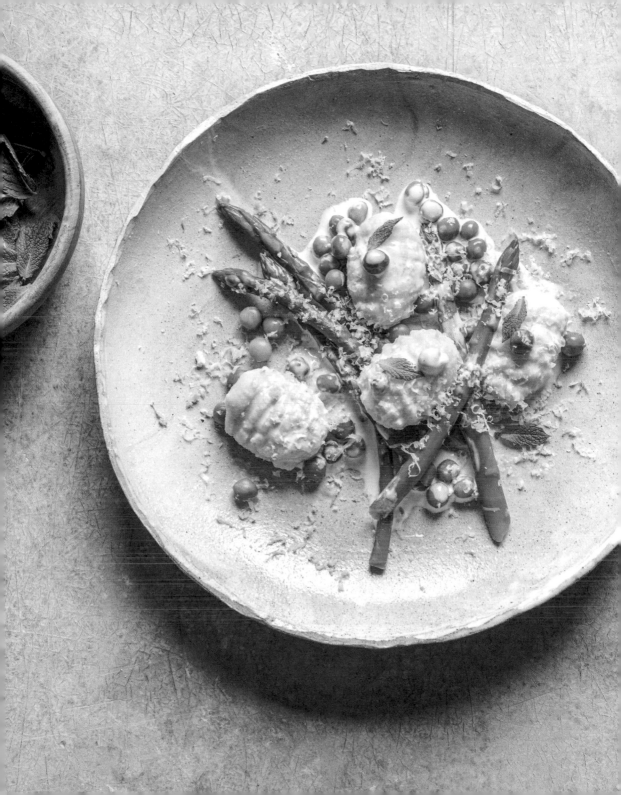

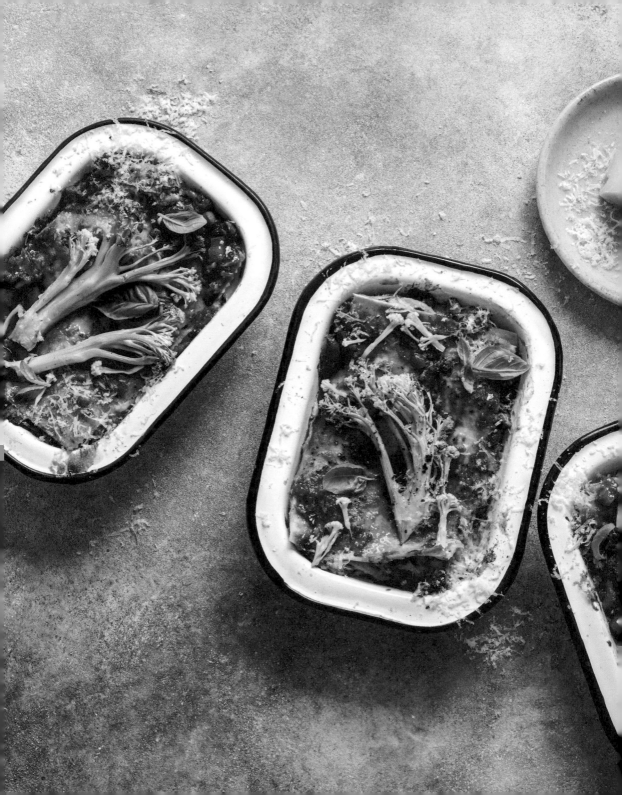

INDIVIDUAL CAULI LASAGNES

Nothing beats a lasagne, and by using fresh pasta it has a more tender finish. With layers of vegetables and mushroom sauce, and topped with cauliflower, it is a perfect dinner party dish.

SERVES 4

3 tablespoons olive oil
½ teaspoon dried chilli flakes/
  hot red pepper flakes
100 g/3½ oz. tenderstem
  cauliflower
300 g/10½ oz. Vegetable Ragù
  (page 94)
150 g/5½ oz. fresh lasagne sheets
100 g/3½ oz. baby spinach
100 g/3½ oz. mixed-colour cherry
  tomatoes, halved
50 g/¾ cup finely grated Parmesan
  or other vegetarian hard cheese

MUSHROOM SAUCE

20 g/1 cup dried porcini mushrooms
2 tablespoons olive oil
4 garlic cloves, crushed
250 g/9 oz. mixed mushrooms,
  sliced
1 sprig rosemary, leaves picked
2 sprigs thyme, leaves picked
500 ml/2 cups crème fraîche
50 g/¾ cup finely grated Parmesan
  or other vegetarian hard cheese
salt and freshly ground black
  pepper

*4 individual lasagne dishes
  (16 x 10 cm/6¼ x 4 inches)*

For the mushroom sauce, cover the dried porcini with boiling water and leave to rehydrate. Heat the olive oil in a pan, add the garlic and cook for 1 minute, then add the mixed mushrooms, herbs and a pinch of salt and pepper. Cook until just starting to colour, stirring regularly. Add the porcini and soaking liquor. Leave to bubble and cook away, then turn the heat down to low, stir in the crème fraîche and cook gently for a few minutes. Remove from the heat, stir in the Parmesan or other hard cheese and set aside.

Preheat the oven to 160°C (325°F) Gas 3.

In a frying pan/skillet, heat the olive oil and the chilli flakes/hot red pepper flakes. Season the cauliflower and add to the pan – there is no need to cook it through, just fry until it has browned nicely on each side. Set aside.

Place a few spoonfuls of the vegetable ragù into each lasagne dish. Top with a fresh lasagne sheet (cut to size), some mushroom sauce, some spinach, another lasagne sheet, the halved cherry tomatoes and another lasagne sheet, and finish with the remaining ragù and the final amount of mushroom sauce. Top with grated Parmesan or other hard cheese and the tenderstem cauliflower, and bake in the preheated oven for 40 minutes until lightly browned on top and the sauce is bubbling.

CAULIFLOWER BROWNIES WITH SALTED COCONUT CARAMEL SAUCE

These healthier brownies are soft and chewy as good brownies should be. The warm coconut caramel sauce is a delicious bonus.

MAKES 16 BROWNIES

350 g/12 oz. cauliflower, leaves and core removed, cut into florets
170 g/1 cup Medjool dates, stones removed
1 teaspoon vanilla bean paste
2 tablespoons espresso coffee
3 tablespoons maple syrup
140 g/1 cup white spelt flour
70 g/generous ¹/₂ cup hazelnuts, ground, plus extra to garnish
50 g/¹/₂ cup unsweetened cocoa powder
¹/₂ tablespoon ground flaxseeds/linseeds
60 g/generous ¹/₃ cup dark/bittersweet chocolate chips
coconut chips, to garnish (optional)

SALTED CARAMEL SAUCE

400-ml/14 fl.-oz. can coconut milk
150 g/5¹/₂ oz. coconut sugar
1 teaspoon vanilla extract
1 tablespoon coconut oil
¹/₂ teaspoon sea salt

20-cm/8-inch square cake pan, greased and lined

Preheat the oven to 180°C (350°F) Gas 4.

First, make the caramel by bringing the coconut milk and coconut sugar to the boil in a pan over a medium-high heat. Reduce the heat to medium-low and then, stirring occasionally, continue to simmer for about 30 minutes, or until the mixture becomes thick and syrupy. Remove from the heat and vigorously stir in the vanilla, coconut oil and salt. Transfer to a glass jar or container and put in the freezer for about an hour, or until the mixture thickens.

Place a colander over a pan of simmering water. Add the cauliflower florets and cover with a lid. Steam for 20 minutes or until tender, then leave to cool. Put the cauliflower in a blender and blitz with the dates, vanilla paste, coffee and maple syrup.

In a bowl, combine the flour, ground hazelnuts, cocoa powder and flaxseeds/linseeds. Stir in the cauliflower mixture until combined. Fold in the chocolate chips and spoon into the lined cake pan. Bake for 20 minutes, until the brownies feel firm to the touch. Remove from the oven and leave to cool in the pan. Cut into squares and drizzle with the caramel sauce to serve. Garnish with extra hazelnuts and coconut chips, if you like.

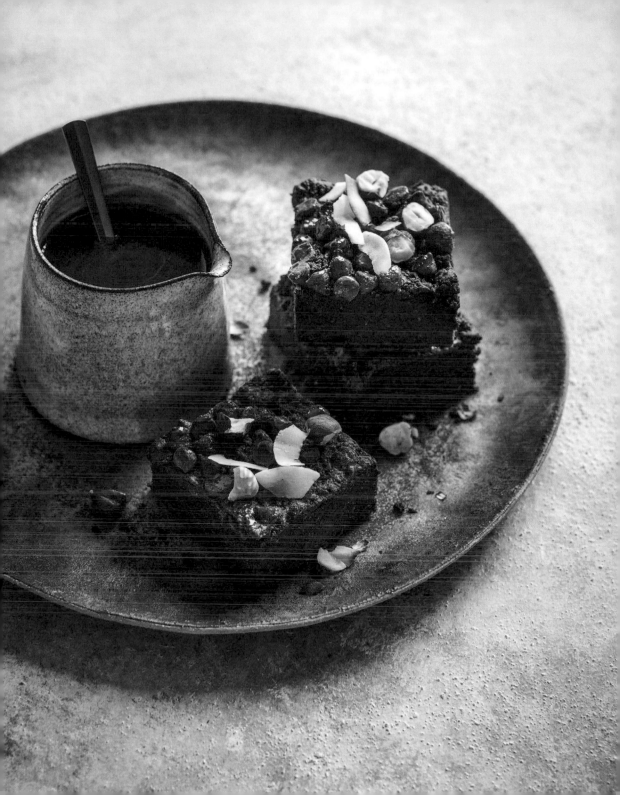

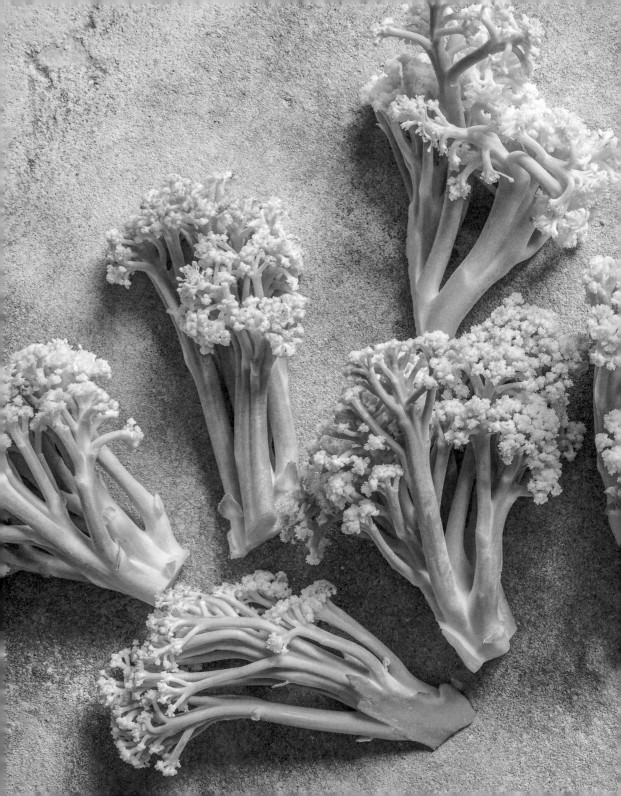

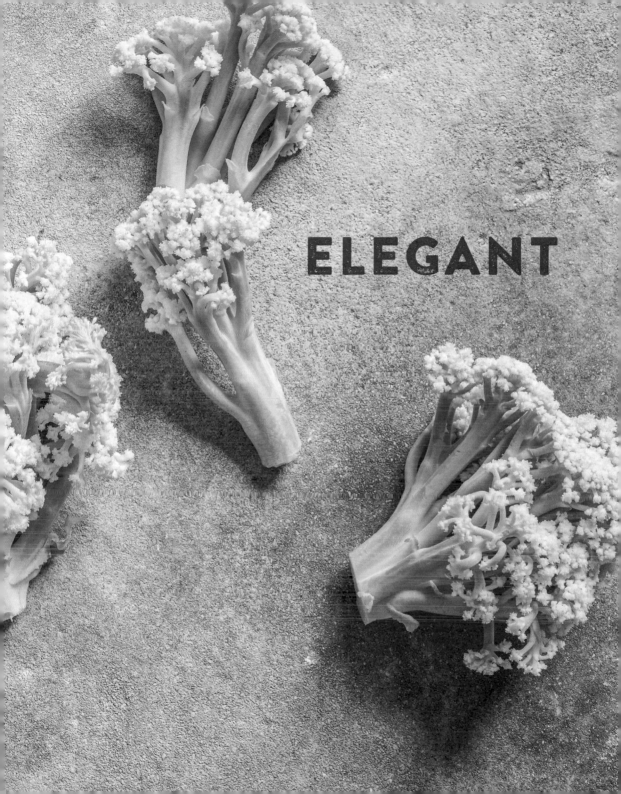

ELEGANT

ARANCINI-STUFFED COURGETTE FLOWERS WITH LEMON & BASIL DIP

This is the perfect way to use up your leftover risotto when courgette/zucchini flowers are in season. Alternatively, simply breadcrumb and fry the risotto balls on their own to make arancini balls.

SERVES 4 (MAKES 16)

½ portion of Cauliflower Risotto without the kale (page 79)
8 courgette/zucchini flowers
vegetable oil, for deep-frying
lemon wedges, to serve

FILLING

2 tablespoons cornflour/cornstarch
small handful of fresh basil, leaves picked and finely chopped
30 g/¼ cup pine nuts, toasted
150 g/5½ oz. mozzarella
40 g/⅓ cup finely grated Parmesan or other vegetarian hard cheese
1 tablespoon sun-dried tomatoes, chopped
grated zest of ½ lemon
salt and freshly ground black pepper

CRISPY COATING

100 g/¾ cup plain/all-purpose flour
2 UK large/US extra-large eggs
200 g/2½ cups dried breadcrumbs

LEMON & BASIL DIP

100 g/scant ½ cup mayonnaise
100 g/scant ½ cup Greek yogurt
grated zest of 1 lemon
2 fresh basil sprigs, leaves picked and chopped

Prepare the cauliflower risotto following the instructions on page 79 and leave to cool, then chill in the fridge.

Mix together the filling ingredients with salt and pepper to taste in a bowl until evenly combined. Scoop a portion of the cooled risotto into your hand and then spoon 1 tablespoon of the filling mixture into the centre and wrap the risotto around it to seal completely. Repeat with the remaining risotto and filling. Stuff each courgette/zucchini flower with a stuffed risotto ball and gently twist the flowers to seal.

Place the flour, beaten eggs and breadcrumbs each into separate shallow bowls. Carefully dip a courgette/zucchini flower into the flour, then the egg, and finally the breadcrumbs, ensuring a complete coating. Set aside and repeat for the rest of the batch.

Heat the oil in a large, heavy-based pan or deep-fat fryer to 180°C (350°F). You can test by dropping a breadcrumb into the hot oil, if it sizzles and rises to the top the oil is ready.

Carefully lower the stuffed courgette/zucchini flowers into the hot oil with a slotted spoon and deep-fry in batches of 2–3 for 8 minutes or until golden and crispy. Transfer to a double layer of paper towels to drain as they are ready.

For the lemon and basil dip, mix the mayonnaise, yogurt, lemon zest and basil together. Serve the courgette/zucchini flowers with the dip and lemon wedges for squeezing over.

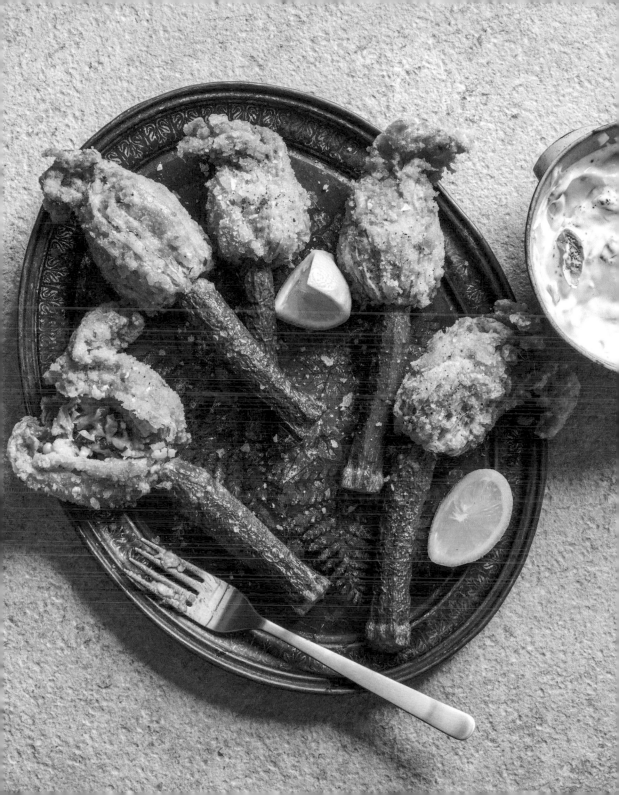

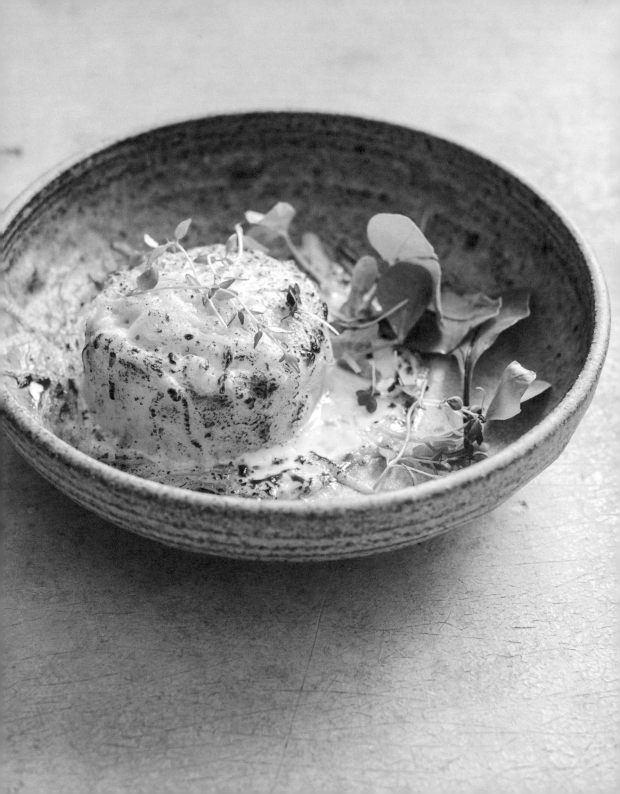

DOUBLE-BAKED CAULIFLOWER SOUFFLÉS

A classic, elegant and impressive way to wow your guests. These can be prepared and baked the first time, then chilled overnight and baked for the second time the next day. Serve with a lovely green side salad.

MAKES 6

200 g/7 oz. cauliflower, cut into florets

1 leek, finely chopped (white part only)

1 tablespoon Dijon mustard

1 onion, finely chopped

1 bay leaf

2 sprigs thyme, plus extra to garnish

350 ml/1½ cups full-fat/whole milk

80 g/¾ stick unsalted butter

120 g/scant 1 cup plain/all-purpose flour

4 eggs, separated

300 ml/1¼ cups double/heavy cream

2 tablespoons finely snipped chives

140 g/1½ cups mixed grated Gruyère and Cheddar

salt and freshly ground black pepper

salad leaves, to serve

6 x 250-ml/9-fl oz ramekins, greased

Preheat the oven to 180°C (350°F) Gas 4.

Place the cauliflower, leek, mustard, onion, bay leaf, thyme and milk in a saucepan over a medium heat. Bring to a simmer, then reduce the heat to low and cook, partially covered, for 8–10 minutes until the cauliflower is tender. Strain, reserving the milk. Discard the herbs.

Melt the butter in another saucepan over a low heat. Add the flour and cook, stirring, for 2–3 minutes. Gradually whisk in the reserved milk. Cook for 2–3 minutes until thickened.

Whisk in the egg yolks, 125 ml/½ cup of the cream and half the mixed cheese. Remove from the heat and set aside.

Blend the cauliflower, leek and onion in a food processor until smooth. Add the sauce and pulse to combine. Season.

In a bowl, using electric beaters, whisk the egg whites to stiff peaks. Fold one-quarter of the egg whites and the chives into the cauliflower mixture to loosen, then gently fold in the remainder. Divide among the prepared ramekins. Place in a deep baking pan and fill with enough boiling water to come halfway up the sides of the ramekins. Bake in the preheated oven for 20 minutes or until puffed and golden.

Remove from the pan and cool slightly, then turn out the soufflés into an oven-proof dish. Pour the remaining cream over the soufflés and scatter with the remaining cheese. Bake for a further 10–15 minutes until risen and bubbling. Serve with salad leaves and extra thyme sprigs, to garnish.

BLACKENED CAULIFLOWER WITH BEETROOT HUMMUS & FIG SALAD

This spice mix is a great go-to blend. A deep flavour is achieved here by topping ghee with the spice mix and searing the cauli until very dark.

SERVES 4

2 heads of cauliflower, rinsed
    and patted dry, each sliced into
    4 steaks, 4 cm/1½ inches thick
2 tablespoons ghee, melted
fresh figs, salad leaves and balsamic
    reduction, to serve

BLACKENED SPICE MIX

2 tablespoons paprika
1 teaspoon cayenne pepper
1 teaspoon onion powder
1 teaspoon garlic powder
1 teaspoon salt
¼ teaspoon ground black pepper
1 teaspoon dried oregano
1 teaspoon coriander seeds, crushed
1 teaspoon dried thyme

BEETROOT/BEET HUMMUS

400-g/14-oz. can chickpeas, drained
250 g/9 oz. cooked beetroot/beets
grated zest and freshly squeezed
    juice of 2 lemons
2 garlic cloves, crushed
4 tablespoons tahini
1 teaspoon ground cumin
½ teaspoon ground coriander
2 tablespoons olive oil (optional)
salt and freshly ground black pepper

For the blackened cauliflower, preheat the oven to 200°C (400°F) Gas 6. Heat up a griddle/grill pan until piping hot.

Mix all the blackened spice mix spices together in a bowl. Brush the cauliflower steaks on both sides with melted ghee and rub with the spice mixture. Char the steaks in the hot griddle/grill pan on each side for a few minutes to colour them, then place on a lined baking sheet.

Bake in the preheated oven for 15 minutes. The cauliflower should be quite dark on the outside but tender on the inside.

Meanwhile, for the beetroot/beet hummus, drain the chickpeas into a bowl (keeping the liquid, which you will use later). Cut the beetroot/beets roughly into cubes. Place the chickpeas, beetroot/beets and lemon zest and juice into a blender or food processor. Add the garlic, followed by the tahini, cumin, coriander and olive oil, if using. Blitz to a smooth paste, then gradually add some of the chickpea liquid, until the desired consistency is reached. Season generously with salt and pepper to your own taste.

Remove the cauliflower steaks from the oven and place on a platter on a bed of the beetroot/beet hummus. Scatter with figs and salad leaves and finish with a drizzle of balsamic reduction.

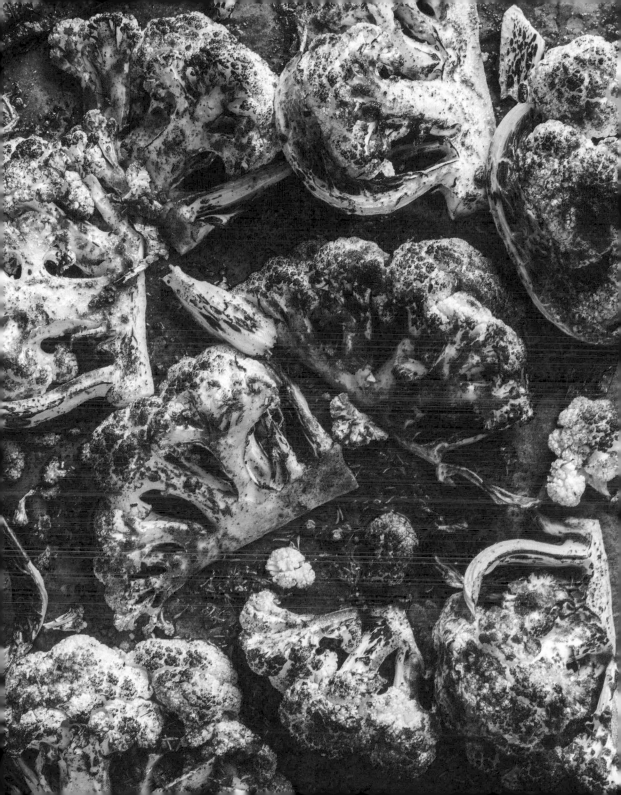

CHARRED CAULIFLOWER Ⓥ

This versatile recipe is great on its own as a side, or mixed through the three salads on these pages. The cauliflower should be charred on the outside and tender inside.

SERVES 4

1 tablespoon ground coriander
1 tablespoon ground cumin
1 tablespoon paprika
½ teaspoon ground ginger
1 teaspoon garlic powder
1 teaspoon salt
1 teaspoon freshly ground black pepper
2 tablespoons olive oil, plus extra
   for brushing
1 cauliflower, cut into wedges

Combine the spices, salt, pepper and oil and set aside. Preheat the grill/broiler to medium. Brush a fresh layer of olive oil onto the cauliflower and sprinkle with the spice mix.

Place the cauliflower wedges directly on the grill/broiler rack and cook until lightly charred, about 5–8 minutes.

Flip and lightly char the other side for the same time.

CAULIFLOWER & QUINOA WITH LIME YOGURT DRESSING

The beauty of this dish is the combination of earthy flavours and tart, creamy dressing.

SERVES 4

1 tablespoon olive oil
150 g/5½ oz. cooked multicoloured quinoa
1 portion of Charred Cauliflower (see left)
80 g/g1 cup flaked/slivered almonds, toasted
60 g/2 oz. fresh coriander, leaves picked
50 g/1¾ oz. fresh mint, leaves picked
50 g/1¾ oz. fresh flat-leaf parsley, leaves
   picked
20 g/¾ oz. fresh dill, roughly chopped
1 teaspoon toasted nigella seeds
lime halves, to serve (optional)

DRESSING

180 g/generous ¾ cup Greek-style yogurt
1 garlic clove, crushed
finely grated zest and juice of 1 lime,
   or to taste
salt and freshly ground black pepper

Add the olive oil to a large frying pan/skillet over a low-medium heat. Add the quinoa and gently toast, stirring, for 3–5 minutes until crisp.

Combine the dressing ingredients in a bowl and season to taste.

Spoon the yogurt dressing onto plates and top with the cauliflower. Scatter with toasted flaked/slivered almonds, quinoa, the herbs and nigella seeds. Squeeze over lime juice and serve.

MIXED BEAN & CAULIFLOWER SALAD Ⓥ

I always have frozen edamame beans, a can of mixed beans and green beans in the fridge as a base for this simple salad.

SERVES 4

1 portion of Charred Cauliflower (see left)
400-g/14-oz can mixed beans, drained and rinsed
200 g/7 oz. fine green beans, blanched
100 g/3¹/₂ oz. edamame beans, blanched
¹/₂ head radicchio, leaves coarsely torn
1 baby fennel bulb, thinly shaved on a mandoline, fronds reserved
40 g/1¹/₂ cups coarsely chopped flat-leaf parsley
2 golden shallots, thinly sliced
¹/₂ garlic clove, finely chopped
50 ml/3¹/₂ tablespoons extra-virgin olive oil
25 ml/1¹/₂ tablespoons apple cider vinegar, or to taste
freshly squeezed juice of 1 lemon

Add the cauliflower to a bowl along with all the beans, the radicchio, fennel, parsley, shallots and garlic. Toss well, then add the extra-virgin olive oil, vinegar and lemon juice and toss to coat. Scatter with fennel fronds and serve.

CAULIFLOWER, FARRO, ENDIVE & BLUE CHEESE SALAD

When cherries are in season I love them in this salad. Roasted grapes with a drizzle of honey make a great autumnal alternative.

SERVES 4

2 dessert apples, cored and sliced
100 g/²/₃ cup cherries, pitted and halved
200 g/7 oz. farro, cooked and cooled
2 endive heads, leaves picked
1 portion of Charred Cauliflower (see left)
200 g/7 oz. blue cheese, crumbled
50 g/¹/₂ cup chopped walnuts

DRESSING

5 tablespoons apple cider vinegar
2 tablespoons olive or rapeseed oil
little drizzle of runny honey
salt and freshly ground black pepper

Make the dressing by whisking the vinegar, olive or rapeseed oil and honey with some salt and pepper.

In a bowl, pour the dressing over the sliced apple, then gently mix in the halved cherries, cooked farro and endives.

Serve on a platter with the charred cauliflower and finish with the blue cheese and walnuts sprinkled over.

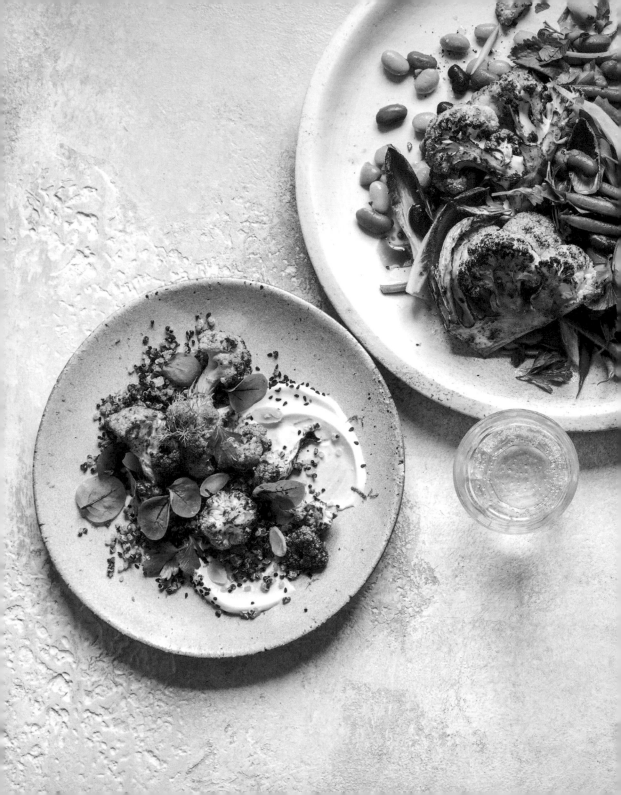

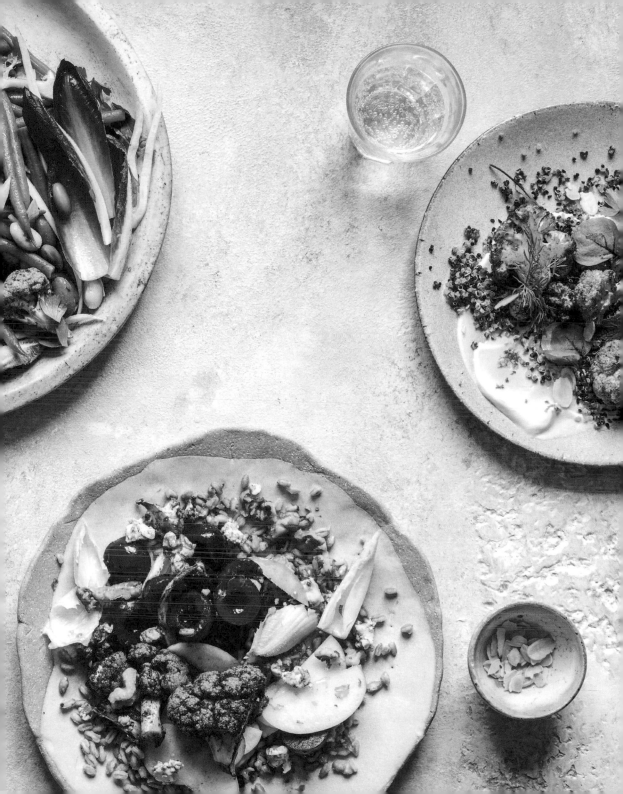

CAULIFLOWER TORTELLINI IN SIMPLE BROTH

An elegant and light pasta dish. Perfect as an appetizer or as a smaller portion for a light main.

SERVES 4

PASTA
2 eggs whisked together with 4 egg yolks
300 g/2¼ cups oo pasta flour mixed with a pinch of salt, plus extra for dusting
semolina flour, for dusting
salt

FILLING
15 g/1 tablespoon butter
1 tablespoon vegetable oil
1 cauliflower, finely chopped
6 tablespoons ricotta
6 tablespoons grated Parmesan or other vegetarian hard cheese, plus extra to serve (optional)
100 g/scant ½ cup mascarpone
salt and freshly ground black pepper

SIMPLE BROTH
2 tablespoons olive oil
2 leeks, halved lengthways, and chopped
1.2 litres/quarts vegetable stock
handful of basil, leaves picked
handful of dill, leaves picked

pasta machine

Gradually stir the egg mixture into the flour in a mixing bowl. Turn the dough out onto a floured surface and knead until smooth. Wrap in clingfilm/plastic wrap and chill.

Meanwhile, for the filling, melt the butter and oil in a pan. Add the cauliflower, season and sauté until golden, about 7 minutes. Add 3 tablespoons water, cover and simmer until tender, about 5 minutes. Uncover and cook until dry, about 3 minutes. Cool completely. Blend the ricotta, Parmesan or other hard cheese and mascarpone in a food processor. Add the cauliflower and blend until smooth. Season.

To form the tortellini, take one-quarter of the pasta dough (keep the rest covered) and feed it through the widest setting on a pasta machine. Then fold it into three, give the dough a quarter turn and feed through the machine again. Repeat once more, then continue to pass the dough through the machine, narrowing the rollers each time. On the narrowest setting, feed the sheet through twice.

Place teaspoons of the filling 4 cm/1½ inches apart on one half of the sheet. Pat water around each blob. Fold the other half of the pasta sheet over the fillings and squeeze around, to remove any air pockets. Cut between each tortellini, then pinch the edges to seal. Repeat with remaining dough and filling.

For the broth, heat the oil in a pan and cook the leeks over a low heat for 5–8 minutes until softened. Add the stock and simmer for 10 minutes, then add the tortellini and simmer until cooked. Stir in the herbs and serve with extra cheese.

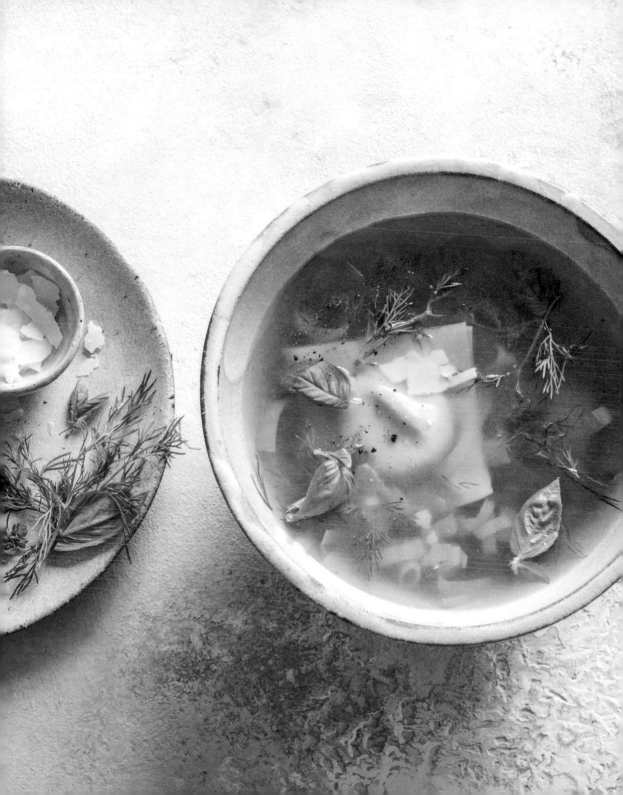

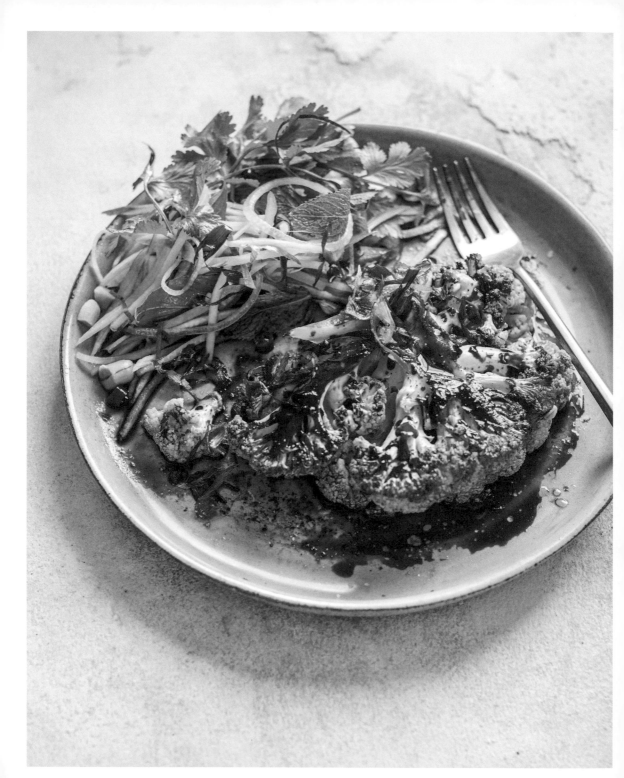

UMAMI CAULIFLOWER STEAKS WITH CRISPY LEEKS

Umami is often described as the ultimate savoury fifth taste. When I am feeling like something a little meaty, this cauliflower dish does the trick.

SERVES 4

4 tablespoons flavourless oil
2 heads of cauliflower, rinsed
    and patted dry, each sliced into
    4 steaks, 4 cm/1¹/₂ inches thick
Asian-style salad, to serve

UMAMI SAUCE

2 tablespoons liquid aminos
1 tablespoon maple syrup
2 garlic cloves, crushed
4-cm/1¹/₂-inch piece ginger, grated
1 teaspoon tomato purée/paste
¹/₄ teaspoon black pepper
2 tablespoons red miso paste,
    blended with water to loosen
2 teaspoons lemon juice
1 tablespoon tamari or soy sauce
freshly squeezed juice of ¹/₂ lime
1 tablespoon black vinegar

CRISPY LEEKS

1 leek
200 ml/scant 1 cup flavourless oil
salt

DRESSING

1 chilli/chile, thinly sliced
freshly squeezed juice of 2 limes
1 tablespoon soy sauce
1 tablespoon palm sugar
3 tablespoons flavourless oil

Preheat the oven to 180°C (350°F) Gas 4. Place a large baking sheet on the middle oven shelf.

Mix together the umami sauce ingredients and set aside.

Place a frying pan/skillet over a medium-high heat and coat with 2 tablespoons of the olive oil. When the pan is smoking, add one steak into the hot oil at a time. Sear on each side for 2 minutes. Repeat with the other steaks, adding oil as needed. Arrange the seared steaks on the preheated baking sheet. Brush with the umami sauce and bake in the oven, basting every 10 minutes, for 25–30 minutes.

Meanwhile, for the crispy leeks, trim off the dark green parts, then thinly slice the white and light green parts of the leek into long julienne strips. Rinse, drain and pat dry.

In a small saucepan heat the oil over a medium-high heat (it should reach a depth of about 2.5 cm/1 inch) until it's between 160–175°C (325–350°F) on a thermometer. Reduce the heat a little to keep the temperature steady. Add a small handful of the leeks to the oil. Fry the leeks, stirring often with a metal slotted spoon, until the oil is barely bubbling and the leeks are light golden brown, 1–3 minutes. Let the oil come back to temperature before frying the next batch. Drain on paper towels. Sprinkle lightly with salt while still hot. Let cool to room temperature.

Mix together the dressing ingredients and serve the steaks with Asian-style salad, drizzled with the cooking juices and dressing and topped with the crispy leeks.

GRATIN DE CHOU-FLEUR

A delicious alternative to a carb-filled potato gratin, yet still sublimely indulgent and comforting.

SERVES 6

½ cauliflower, cut into florets
2 courgettes/zucchini, thinly sliced
   on an angle
100 g/3½ oz. Brussels sprouts,
   thinly sliced
70 g/5 tablespoons butter
40 g/5 tablespoons plain/
   all-purpose flour
1 litre/quart full-fat/whole milk
200 g/scant 2 cups grated Gruyère
   cheese
1 teaspoon freshly chopped thyme
½ teaspoon freshly grated nutmeg
50 g/⅔ cup dried breadcrumbs
salt and freshly ground black
   pepper

baking dish, buttered

Preheat the oven to 190°C (375°F) Gas 5.

Steam the cauliflower in a large pot of boiling water fitted with a steamer basket for 5–7 minutes, until the florets are just tender. Rinse them in cold water, drain, and arrange them in a single layer in the buttered dish. Add the raw sliced courgettes/zucchini and sprouts.

In a large saucepan over a medium heat, melt the butter and whisk in the flour until it forms a smooth paste. Continue whisking and cook for about 2 minutes, then gradually add the milk, a little at a time. Add half the cheese and stir until melted. Continue whisking and cook until the sauce is heated through, smooth and thickened. Remove from the heat and season with salt, the thyme and nutmeg.

Pour 500 ml/2 cups of the béchamel sauce over the cauliflower, courgettes/zucchini and sprouts, and gently toss the florets to make sure they are thoroughly coated with the sauce. Bake the gratin, uncovered, in the preheated oven for 15 minutes.

Stir together the remaining grated Gruyère cheese and the breadcrumbs and sprinkle them over the gratin.

Bake it for an additional 10–15 minutes, until the gratin is hot and bubbly and the cheese is melted and browned. Sprinkle the surface of the baked gratin with black pepper and serve hot.

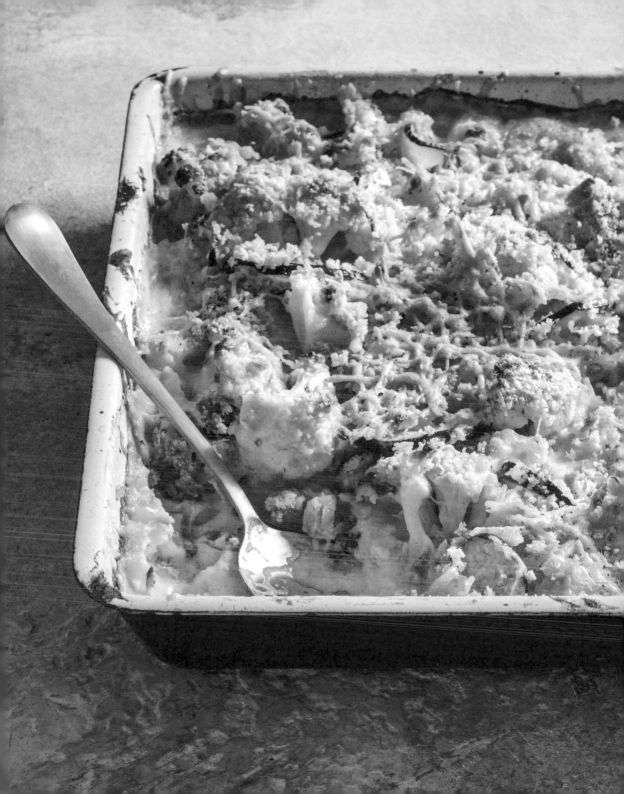

INDEX

ACKNOWLEDGEMENTS

Thank you to Mowie Kay for the perfect photography and just being fabulous. The lovely Olivia Wardle for wonderful props, always. Evangeline Hardbury for tasting and testing the recipes and assisting me on the shoot – your opinion and skill are invaluable. Anna Hiddleston, thank you for testing recipes and being by my side – a true pleasure to be around. Claudia Lazarus – for sharing your passion for food and assisting the team on set. At Ryland Peters & Small, thank you to Sonya Nathoo – it is always an absolute pleasure to work with you – thank you is not enough. Alice Sambrook and Kate Reeves-Brown, you do all the hard work – thank you for editing and keeping me on track. Leslie Harrington and Julia Charles, thank you for always being available, your guidance and encouragement. Thank you to my publisher Cindy Richards, for giving me the opportunity to work on such a lovely project with a great team. Finally, thank you to my friends and family the world over!

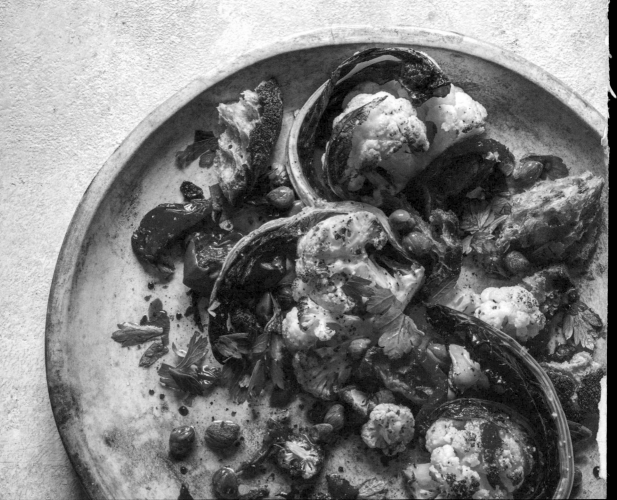